The Art & Practice of

SPIRITUAL HERBALISM

TRANSFORM, HEAL, & REMEMBER *with the* POWER *of* PLANTS *and* ANCESTRAL MEDICINE

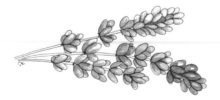

KAREN M. ROSE

Creator of *Sacred Vibes Apothecary*

FAIR WINDS

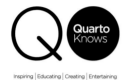

Inspiring | Educating | Creating | Entertaining

Brimming with creative inspiration, how-to projects, and useful information to enrich your everyday life, Quarto Knows is a favorite destination for those pursuing their interests and passions. Visit our site and dig deeper with our books into your area of interest: Quarto Creates, Quarto Cooks, Quarto Homes, Quarto Lives, Quarto Drives, Quarto Explores, Quarto Gifts, or Quarto Kids.

First Published in 2022 by Fair Winds Press, an imprint of The Quarto Group,
100 Cummings Center, Suite 265-D, Beverly, MA 01915, USA.
T (978) 282-9590 F (978) 283-2742 QuartoKnows.com

Fair Winds Press titles are also available at discount for retail, wholesale, promotional, and bulk purchase. For details, contact the Special Sales Manager by email at specialsales@quarto.com or by mail at The Quarto Group, Attn: Special Sales Manager, 100 Cummings Center, Suite 265-D, Beverly, MA 01915, USA.

25 24 23 22 21   1 2 3 4 5

ISBN: 978-0-7603-7179-4

Digital edition published in 2022
eISBN: 978-0-7603-7180-0

Library of Congress Cataloging-in-Publication Data available

Design and Page Layout: Tanya Jacobson, jcbsn.co
Photography: JazzShoots, JazzShoots.com
Illustration: Elayna Speight, Inked Designs, ThinkInkedDesigns.com, @thinkinkedart

Printed in China

The information in this book is for educational purposes only. It is not intended to replace the advice of a physician or medical practitioner. Please see your health-care provider before beginning any new health program.

DEDICATION

*I am grateful to have found my
children and coconspirators again:
Lauren, Zion, and Shiloh.*

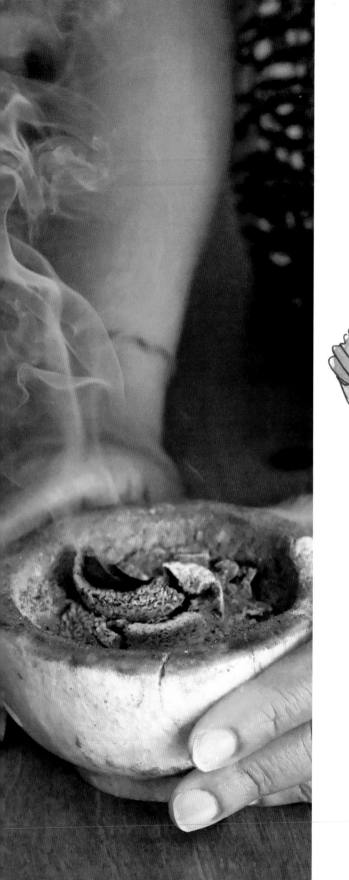
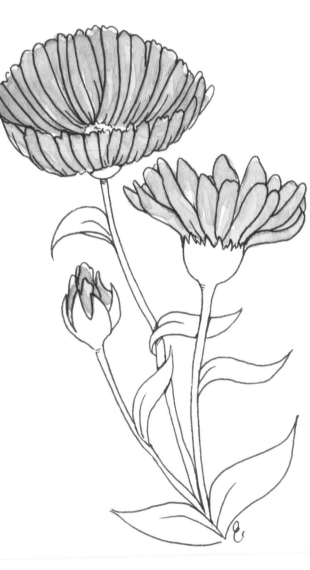

CONTENTS

INTRODUCTION: SPIRITUAL HERBALISM

————

I am a first-generation immigrant whose healing practice reflects my grandmother's teachings in Guyana. She was a medicine holder and plant healer. Today I continue my grandmother's legacy as a healer and herbalist.

As a Black, indigenous, young herbalist in the West, it was challenging to see where I fit in. How do you value and measure knowledge held in the body, innate ancestral knowing? For many years I felt my ancestral knowledge was devalued by my herbal community. Western herbalism practitioners lack reverence for, and have colonized many indigenous ancestral traditions. While they exploit resources and modalities, they are often unwilling to uplift indigenous practitioners and healers.

Growing up in Essequibo, Guyana, a small village along the Atlantic Ocean's coast, we relied on our community to support our physical and spiritual healing. Everyone in the small village where I grew up knew which plants help with which ailments. When something was beyond what we could do, we visited the community's healers. I grew up visiting local healers each time I was sick, because we would have to travel to the city to see a doctor. We achieved wellness as varied as the healers themselves through plants, chants, prayers, laying of hands, and physical manipulation.

My family lost its connection to plants when we emigrated to the United States, as we tried to assimilate to this land's culture. We went to doctors instead of healers. My conscious return to plants began more than two decades ago with the birth of my daughter, Lauren. I used plants to heal her, and I teach her this knowledge, as my grandmother taught me.

My ancestors are from Ghana, the Congo, China, and India. I bring their indigenous practices forward in my work today. In my spiritual herbalism program, I teach what I've learned in my studies and observed as a youth. My healing work encompasses plants, ancestral practices, and community. This practice brings the Spirits back to herbalism, as it was when our indigenous ancestors walked this world.

The framework for spiritual herbalism is built on a relational vision of health, with the understanding that we cannot heal alone in a vacuum. A healthy relationship with our families, communities, environment, Earth, and Spirit is necessary to heal. We utilize plants consciously and sustainably to heal our spirit and bodies and connect back to the land, our communities, and our ancestors. We uplift our ancestors' teachings, honor and revere their work, and align ourselves with their traditional practices to heal our generations forward and backward.

Plants teach us how to access our resilience, and they are resilient even through the devastation of their environment. For example, ginkgo and birch trees were the first to appear after the nuclear bomb dropped on Hiroshima. So too our ancestral healing knowledge and wisdom survived even the harshest conditions of enslavement and colonization to reach our ears and hearts today. Targeted for extinction and eradication, it springs up with a lushness we could not fathom.

As a descendant of enslaved people and indentured servants, I feel their resilience and traumas coexist in my body. To practice medicine and healing without acknowledgment of these truths is, in effect, malpractice. Our families' history reflects in our bodies and manifests as illnesses, such as heart disease, diabetes, or digestive issues. It can also be the source of extraordinary gifts, such as spiritual sight or clairvoyance, which require physical and spiritual balance.

Plants help us navigate finding harmony by supporting knowledge of the Self, which creates agency and power. Plant medicine turns us inward to witness the Self, reclaim our ancestors' resilience, and fortify our spirits so we can do the work of healing. What we consider hereditary is, in fact, an inherited ancestral spiritual contract, and until we begin the work of ancestral healing, the agreement continues to exist inside our bodies. A spiritual inheritance or hereditary physical response offers us an opportunity to heal beyond ourselves, healing lineages.

The body yearns to return to ancestral wisdom and connection. And the body becomes a great wake-up call when disharmony enters to change our pattern of thinking and living. These issues come up so they can guide us to wholeness and integration. If you are here, the ancestors chose you to begin this vital work. This book will guide you through this process of self-healing and ultimately healing past and future generations. Know that you are enough and step forward.

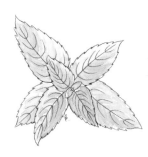

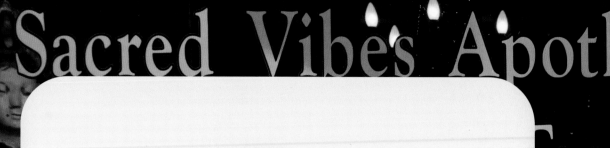

Building a Courageous Heart

CIRCULATORY HEALTH

——

Our heart is a muscle and, if we ignore it, it becomes silent and atrophied. By the time we see the physical signs of our hearts hardening, we have already been in the practice of denying our hearts for some time.

In indigenous healing cultures, heart problems signal discontent and unhappiness. Discontent emerges when we make all of our decisions from a rational or logical place. Making decisions from our heads and not our hearts leads to disconnection. Each time we override what we feel in our hearts with logic and reason, our hearts shrink more.

Suppressing our deepest emotions suppresses our inner light and holds our joy prisoner. How have we been complicit in dimming our light? In what ways have we blocked our peace and happiness by withholding our light?

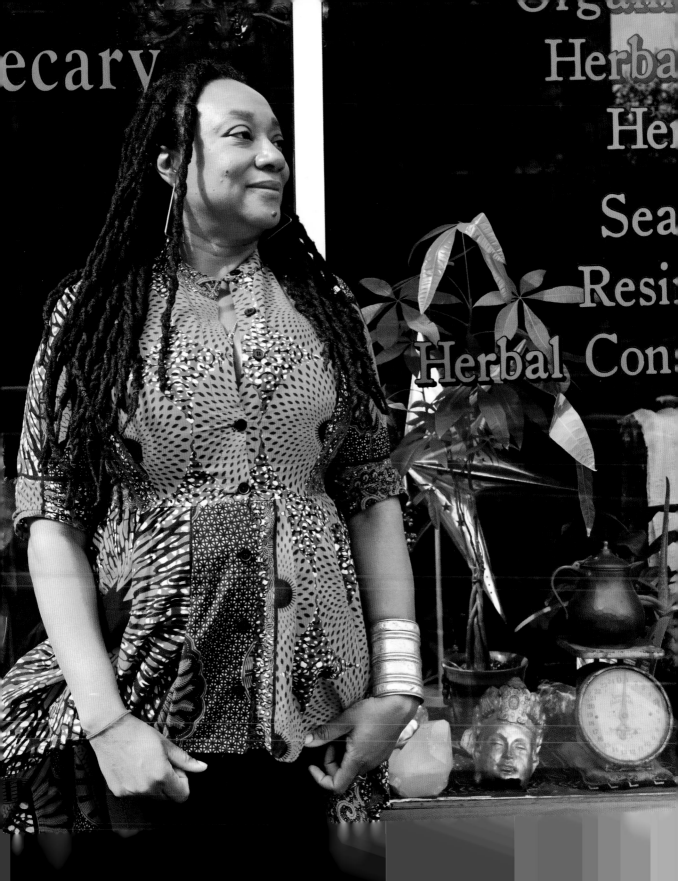

There may have been a wound that led us to ignore our hearts. As children or young people, we may have had to harden to survive. Over time a detached, closed heart shows up in our bodies as a circulatory system, blood vessel, or heart issue. As adults it is up to us to connect with, heal, and build a courageous and resilient heart. Healing work opens a closed heart and encourages reconnection.

Tap into your heart's leadership, listen, and be led by its answers. Wisdom finds a home in our hearts, not our heads. Make it a practice to move fearlessly with what the heart wants. Our lives change when we move from a heart-centered place—meaning we elicit the heart's desires and center them in all our daily decisions. Heart-centeredness can occur all the time, not just when sitting in meditation: It is as simple as listening to the heart, uplifting its value and importance in our life.

A practice that helps me connect to my heart each day is to ask: What does my heart want to eat today? What does my heart want me to wear today? When someone invites me somewhere, does my heart want to go? Then I act accordingly. The more we can tap into the heart's innate wisdom, the more decisions come naturally, as we trust our heart and intuition—this is the path to a heart-centered life.

The Spirit of the Circulatory System

The Sun guides the circulatory system. And just as the Sun is the center and warms each orbiting planet, the heart is our center, pumping blood, oxygen, and warmth to each organ. The Sun, the heart, and the circulatory system remind us to center ourselves and be present in our power, changing the focus from others to ourselves.

The Sun is central to our solar system. We ask people what their Sun sign is when we are trying to determine who they are at their deepest level, their core. Who are you at your core? Are you happy there?

Our hearts and our minds need a balanced relationship. On the Native American Medicine Wheel, the heart sits in the south. This energy is outward and giving. The heart's relationship to giving and receiving is primal in heart health. The heart's whole design is to give and receive. As the heart gets blood from the body, it flows through the chambers, through the lungs to receive oxygen, and back out to nourish the body.

Joy and flow are the lessons of the circulatory system. Disorders or imbalances of the heart, whether physiological or emotional, stem from blocking these two complementary forces from our lives. Do we center the heart? Are we sustained in reciprocal exchanges? Or are we giving in sacrifice, extending ourselves from a place of exhaustion and depletion?

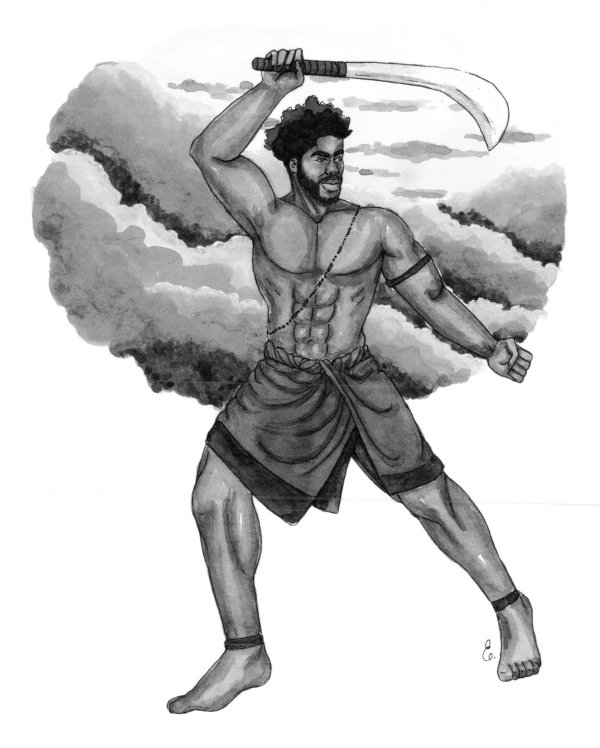

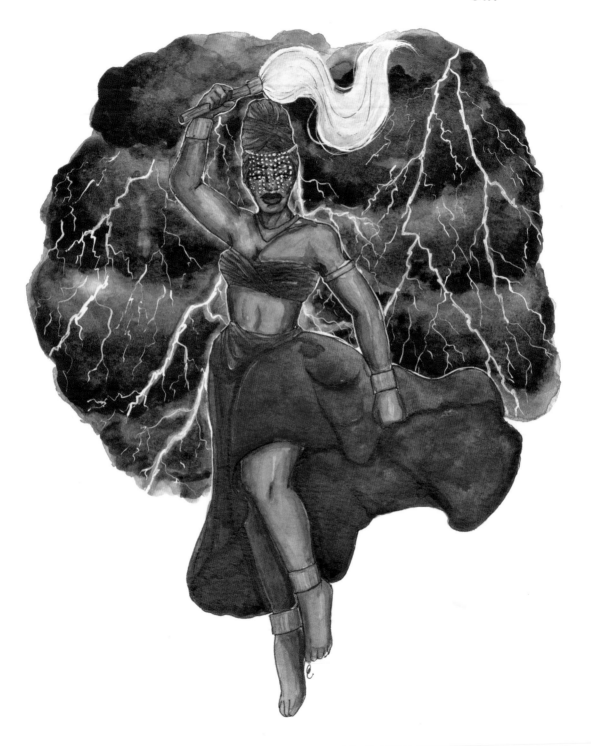

In the African diaspora, the heart is guided by the Sun and the orisha Oggun, and it is coruled by Oya. While Oggun, the orisha of war, may clear the path so blood can flow, Oya is the orisha of winds and change. Oya ushers in needed transitions to elevate our being—and a healthy heart gives us the ability to go with these changes. A trusting heart allows us to surrender control, listen to this spiritual direction, and flow.

The valves in our hearts only open in one direction. There is no going against the circulatory system. When we resist change, our hearts struggle. Trying to go against the heart means fighting our very nature. To begin a fight with Oggun is always a losing battle: Oggun is a courageous warrior and a protector who wields a machete. The heart, like Oggun, has the power to go to war for our entire body. Our heart's machete is love.

Love is life, and we have come to know God is Love. The heart's design is to process love, the highest vibration in this Universe, and an open heart is responsive to that vibration. When we open our hearts freely and center love, our hearts are protected and fierce. It is courageous and wise to walk through this world with our hearts open: A hardened, closed, cold heart cannot receive. Even our ancestral gifts are left unreceived.

As with other muscles in our bodies, building a healthy heart requires stretching and strengthening. Navigating and healing through emotions such as pain, hurt, betrayal, grief, or loss helps us shore up the heart's resilience. These emotions often demand that we stretch our hearts further, and this opening can feel like breaking. Instead it is breaking open to more compassion and empathy than ever before.

The Heart

The circulatory system is composed of the heart, blood, and more than 60,000 miles of blood vessels, which carry blood through the body and back to the heart. Blood circulation is essential to provide our bodies with oxygen and remove our cells' carbon dioxide. The circulatory system is one of the major networks in our body to distribute nutrients and hormones, move our white blood cells, and transport platelets to injury sites to repair damaged tissue. The circulatory system is a system of nourishment, communication, and defense.

The major vessels are the arteries and veins, which are subdivided into arterioles and venules, respectively, eventually becoming capillaries, threadlike vessels that link the arterial and venous systems. As the body uses the oxygen transported by the blood, the blood returns to the heart. Blood passes through the right side of the heart, receives oxygen from the lungs, then passes back through the left side of the heart before being pumped back out to the rest of the body. Arteries carry oxygen-rich blood away from the heart to the body's organs, while veins return blood to the heart to receive oxygen again.

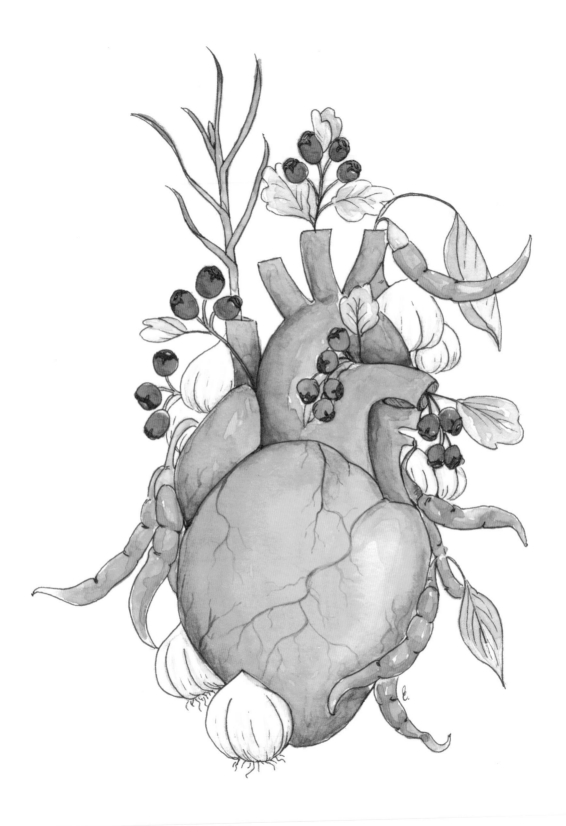

The Art & Practice of SPIRITUAL HERBALISM

Vitality and tone of the circulatory system are fundamental to life and the integration of all parts of the body. If weaknesses and congestion are present, it will profoundly affect the tissues and organs involved. Lack of blood and oxygen can cause damage to tissues or even stop essential functions. Likewise hardened or clogged arteries limit the amount of blood, oxygen, and nutrients available to the body and force our hearts to work harder. Clots or other blockages can cause a stroke or pulmonary embolism. Similarly if waste materials produced by our metabolic processes are not removed, damage to the tissues will result.

High blood pressure is our body's response to the environment and the structural stresses we navigate daily. The body reflects the constant accumulation of stressors and their impact as they become integrated into our daily lives. It is sad to think that we may not even be familiar with how our bodies feel without stress.

High blood pressure can also be the body's response to going against the grain, swimming against the current, and not going with the flow. If we are continually directing everything that goes on around us, we cannot flow. Being a perfectionist reflects on heart health. Trust in your heart, and let it lead you to where you are supposed to be.

In cases of high blood pressure, I remind my clients to center rest. Rest is radical in a world that rewards productivity. Often we are overreaching, overachieving, and overcomplicating our lives instead of just being. In my practice I have seen many people with issues connected to the heart have jobs in leadership or activism roles that lead to the heart's overextension. To heal, the heart takes conscious work to develop new patterns that instill rest, sitting still, and finding and connecting to pleasure instead of constantly pressing forward. I remind my clients of this simple notion, the notion of being.

While high blood pressure may be more common, low blood pressure also indicates that we are not in flow. We are not struggling against it because we don't even jump in. We are fearful, standing on the precipice, not wanting to appear foolish. We are so worried about our next move and the next step that we choose not to engage. That worry smothers the heart's fire as we wait for permission to live our lives.

The heart, like all muscles, wants to be used and nourished. Occasionally we must stretch the heart to help strengthen it. We can do this by moving vigorously enough to raise our heart rate at least three times a week. We also want to be mindful of what we are feeding our hearts. We should limit our intake of fats and salts, particularly when hidden, added as a preservative, or used to make processed foods taste better. Our diet should consist of plenty of fresh fruits, vegetables, whole grains, beans, and peas to reduce our cholesterol levels. If you have concerns about your heart and blood vessels, consider limiting smoking and alcohol intake.

Plants for the Heart

The circulatory system requires fire, and the plants that bring healing are fiery ones, identified with Oggun—cayenne, garlic, and hawthorn. These Mars and Fire plants heal a cold, disconnected heart and breathe life and light back into the body after trauma. Fire plants help us reestablish connections with ourselves. In their own distinct ways, each of these plants connects us to flow and joy and helps us move from a heart-centered place. They are suitable for forgiveness work as they bring back vitality and wholeness to the heart. They stimulate cellular memories and bring forth resilience, allowing for healing while breaking ancestral karmic patterns.

Plants guided by Oggun fortify, protect, and give courage to our childlike hearts. They help us create protection for our hearts from the inside, allowing us to be vulnerable and step forward into our passion.

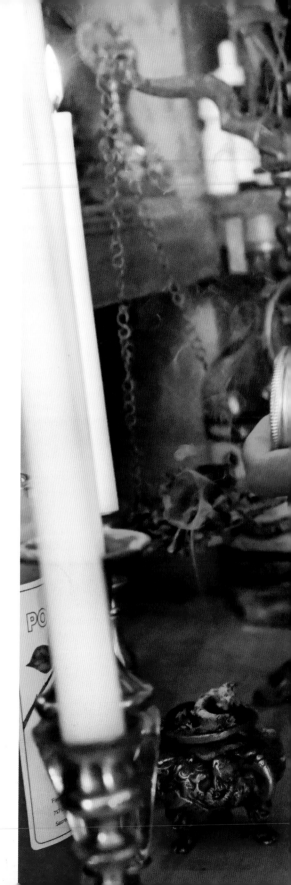

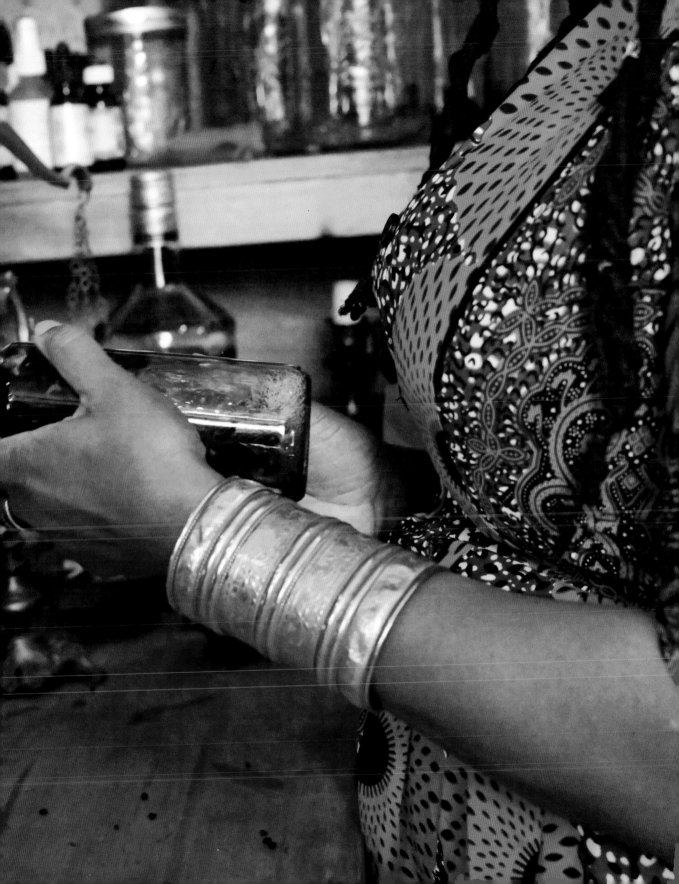

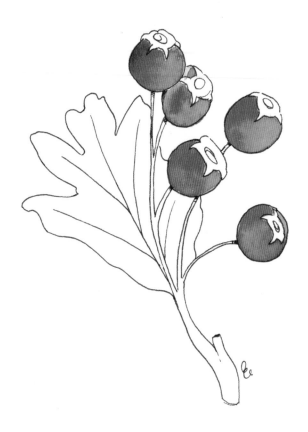

HAWTHORN

Hawthorn's thorns caution us that protection is needed when we move through this world with an open heart. Hawthorn plants have huge thorns with sharp tips that wound the skin, reminding us to be present with our approach to our hearts and the hearts of others. As a plant whose energy is Oggun, it gives us courage and fortifies our hearts. It helps us shield ourselves while still functioning from a heart-centered place. Hawthorn is excellent for someone who needs help with giving and receiving love.

Hawthorn is one of my favorite medicines for heartbreak and sadness, as it helps us grieve and prepare our hearts for the energy of new love, bringing back the heart's passion.

Common Name: Hawthorn

Latin Name: *Crataegus oxyacantha*

Other Names: May Tree, Mayflower, Mayblossom, Thorn, White Thorn

Taxonomy: Rosaceae

Botanical Description: Hawthorn is a small tree with thorns and clusters of fragrant flowers that are white to pink and bloom in May. Dark red berries ripen in the fall.

Native Habitat: England; North Africa; temperate regions of the northern hemisphere

Wildcrafting and Cultivation: Hawthorn's flowers are open for a short time in May. Gather berries when red and ripe in late fall. Grow from seeds in moist, alkaline soil. Trees prefer sun.

Parts Used: Berries, leaves, and flowers

Planetary Influence/Correspondence: Mars, Fire

Energetic Quality: Sour, hot

Pharmacological Constituents: Flavonoids; saponins; coumarin; glycosides; tannins; antioxidants

Ethnobotanical/Historical Use: Hawthorn has a long history in Druid culture. Considered a sacred tree, hawthorn was used in the Maypole ritual to represent fertility, happiness, and hope. Leaves were used in sandwiches, so it was sometimes called "bread and cheese tree."

Actions/Properties: Cardiotonic; regulates heartbeat; vasodilator; diuretic; astringent; normalizer of blood pressure; strengthens heart muscle

Indications: Cardiac weakness and failure; pain; irregular heartbeat; murmurs; enlarged heart; high or low blood pressure; rapid heartbeat; arteriolosclerosis; insomnia; stress; water retention; breathlessness

Contraindications: Work with a doctor to use hawthorn if you are on heart medication, have ulcers, or have colitis.

Methods of Preparation and Dosage

Decoction: Soak a handful of hawthorn berries overnight, and then simmer in 2 cups (475 ml) water in the morning for 25 to 30 minutes. Drink throughout your day.

For Whole-Plant Medicine: Decoct the berries, then add the flowers and leaves. Infuse for an additional 25 minutes.

Tincture: Use 15 to 30 drops of tincture 3 times a day.

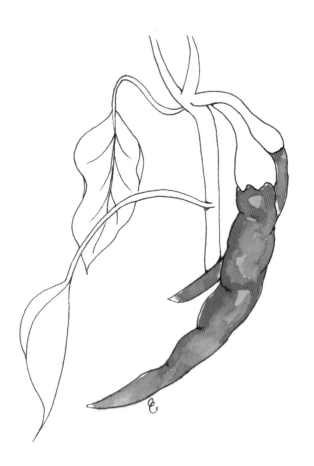

CAYENNE

Cayenne's medicine brings movement and transformation. It is a fast-acting catalyst that is dynamic in waking up body processes. It reawakens cold, disconnected hearts that have been traumatized or frozen. Cayenne can be used for heart attack and shock. It brings its user back to their body and can be helpful for trauma, susto (intense fear/shock/trauma), or soul loss. When events happen that take our breath away and freeze our action, cayenne can allow us to be present, turning energy into action.

Cayenne brings blood, warmth, and energy. It is one of my favorite aphrodisiacs. I have used it with chocolate and hot chocolate to evoke passion. Use cayenne to promote self-love, heat a cold romantic relationship, or remove a creative block.

Scatter cayenne around your door and property to break hexes and release you back to your power. As a plant of Oggun, cayenne courageously strengthens the heart's voice and provides protection and vitality.

Cayenne is an excellent introductory herb to use with people who do not usually use herbal medicine because it is accessible; most homes have cayenne in the spice cabinet.

Common Name: Cayenne

Latin Name: *Capsicum frutescens* or *Capsicum annuum*

Other Names: Red Pepper, Bird Pepper, Fruit of the Sun

Taxonomy: Solanaceae

The Art & Practice of SPIRITUAL HERBALISM

Botanical Description: Cayenne is an annual plant with lancelot leaves and drooping star-shaped flowers. The plant has greenish to yellow fruits, which ripen to yellow or red.

Native Habitat: Tropical Americas; introduced to Europe and India

Wildcrafting and Cultivation: Sow cayenne by seed. It likes full sun. Gather in the summer when fruits ripen.

Parts Used: Fruit

Planetary Influence/Correspondence: Mars, Fire

Energetic Quality: Pungent, hot

Pharmacological Constituents: Capsaicin; alkaloids; flavonoids; ascorbic acid; minerals; sulfur; vitamin A; vitamin B complex; vitamin C; zinc

Ethnobotanical/Historical Use: Cayenne has a long history of use throughout the Americas. The Navajo used it to wean babies. It was one of the four sacred plants in Mexico, along with corn, squash, and beans.

Actions/Properties: Stimulates the circulatory system; diaphoretic; antibacterial; alterative; antispasmodic; carminative; digestive; rubefacient; sialagogue; stimulant; cardiac tonic; anti-inflammatory; anticatarrhal; regulates blood pressure; decongestant; hemostatic.

Indications: First aid remedy for heart attack or shock; poor circulation; poor absorption; fatigue; high or low blood pressure; arthritis; flatulence; intestinal bacterial; varicose veins; high cholesterol; internal or external bleeding; Alzheimer's disease; dementia

Contraindications: Do not inhale cayenne during an asthma attack. Do not use topically on damaged or sensitive skin. Do not use it internally if there are ulcers, inflammation in the digestive tract, IBS, acid reflux, or exposed mucosa. Milk and yogurt are good antidotes for too much cayenne. Purchase organic cayenne powder; conventional is often contaminated with lead oxide.

Methods of Preparation and Dosage

Use with Food: Medicinal dose is ⅛ teaspoon. Use cayenne in food, water, juice, or soup. Stir into a shot glass of apple cider vinegar or grape juice and drink as a heart tonic.

External Uses: For a first aid remedy, sprinkle powdered cayenne on a wound if you cut yourself to stop the bleeding. Rub cayenne-infused oil on swollen joints, the back for back pain, or apply over the womb area for menstrual cramps. During a heart attack or shock, place 1 teaspoon of the dry powder on the tip of the tongue.

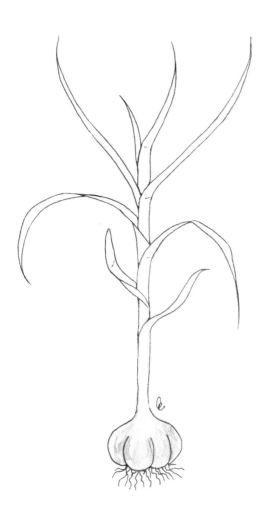

GARLIC

Garlic is strong medicine with a strong lingering aroma. It helps shield us from emotional vampires. It protects our energy and repels harmful energy that may be coming to us. Growing up, my family used garlic skins to protect us spiritually—we would burn them over our babies and in our homes to remove any unwanted energies. Garlic also removes curses from our ancestral lineages, purifying the bloodlines and toxic belief systems.

Most homes already have garlic, which makes for an easy transition to use this plant in healing. Use it to remove unwanted vibrations from old relationships or objects. Garlic is excellent for treating blood impurities and it moves stagnation.

Common Name: Garlic

Latin Name: *Allium sativum*

Other Names: Stinking Rose

Taxonomy: Liliaceae

Botanical Description: Garlic bulbs are composed of individual cloves and white skin. Garlic has long, flat leaves that grow up to 3 feet (1 m) tall and star-shaped white flowers.

Native Habitat: Native to Central Asia; cultivated around the world

Wildcrafting and Cultivation: Gather wild garlic bulbs in spring. Plant from the bulb in the fall. It likes partial sun to shade.

Parts Used: Bulbs

Planetary Influence / Correspondence: Mars, Fire

Energetic Quality: Dry, spicy, hot, yang

Pharmacological Constituents: Allicin; volatile oils

Ethnobotanical/Historical Use: Garlic was used by Greeks, Romans, Chinese, Egyptians, and many other cultures. Egyptians used garlic to increase strength and endurance and to guard against the plague. Around the Mediterranean, grave robbers used thieves' oil, made in part from garlic, to protect against the plague.

Actions/Properties: Adaptogen; alterative; antibiotic; anticoagulant; antifungal; anti-neoplastic; antiseptic; antispasmodic; blood purifier; diaphoretic; digestive; expectorant; rubefacient; stimulant; vulnerary

Indications: Blood impurities, diseases, poisoning, and infections; strep infection, staph infection, high blood pressure, and heart disease; lung disorders, coughs, colds, ear and upper respiratory infections, flu, and candida. Enhances the immune system. Stimulates the lymph system to rid the body of waste and parasites. Garlic is an excellent antibiotic. Use for bacterial vaginosis, respiratory infections, and other bacterial infections.

Contraindications: Do not use garlic with an irritated digestive tract or excess heat conditions such as anger and irritability.

Methods of Preparation and Dosage

Use as Food: Use garlic raw. Garlic loses its medicinal properties when cooked. You can make bruschetta, garlic vinegar, garlic honey, or salad dressing. The standard dosage is 1 clove 3 times a day.

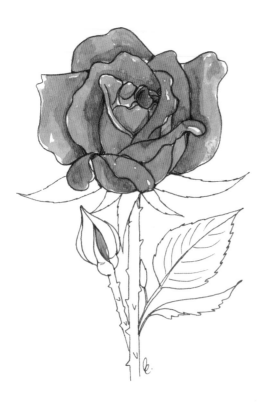

ADDITIONAL PLANTS

Rose *Rosa* spp.

The high-vibration rose is one of the most extraordinary plants. Its aroma and softness are unforgettable. Rose's thorns protect its beauty: Beauty needs protection. This plant reminds us that blooming into our most radiant selves requires protection as a baseline.

As a Venus/Oshun plant, rose connects us to our sensuality and heart, restoring vitality and joy. Rose medicine is needed now, in our revolutionary work of loving the self. It calms the fire of an overused heart, allowing us to hold energy for ourselves and, from there, extend to loving others.

I am a huge fan of rose. It is my namesake. Many ask me whether I changed my name, as herbalists do with rose. My answer is no. I grew into my ancestral name by walking this path as an herbalist. I come for a long line of Roses, who got their name from their enslaver. Like many Black families, we continue to wrestle with this knowledge while embracing our ancestral legacy. I uplift all the ways my ancestors stood in their beauty, joy, and resilience, like a rose. I work with rose medicine often, and each time I touch this plant, I stand in my name, sending healing backward through the lineage to my ancestors.

Rose, with all its beauty, is strong plant medicine. It is antiviral, antidepressant, astringent, aphrodisiac, and anti-inflammatory. It is beneficial for colds, flu, and sore throat. Rose hips, the fruit and seedpod of the plant, are antiseptic, high in vitamin C, nourishing, and can bring down a fever.

Contraindications: Do not use sprayed roses, or hybrid roses without scent or soul.

The Art & Practice of SPIRITUAL HERBALISM

Nettles *Urtica dioica*

Nettles are an excellent introduction to what nourishment can feel like in our bodies. They are packed with vitamins and minerals, and can be used as a daily tonic, giving us vitality. Nettles are fiery by nature. We must be present and attentive when we pick nettles or they will sting us. Nettles demand that we approach with intention, and they teach us how to demand that same presence and respect in our relationships.

This Mars and Fire-guided plant helps us center on self-care first. Only when we are deeply nourished can we share nourishment without self-depletion. The plant has a historical use in exorcism, removing hexes, and stopping gossip. I often refer to nettles as exorcising energies from our bodies: We begin our day with one energy and throughout the day, as we are in contact with others, our entire energy shifts. Nettles help us return to ourselves by removing any energies that are not our own. Drinking nettles fortifies us and shields us from energies that might be seeking a home.

Nettles build our blood's iron and are useful for any hemorrhaging in the body, including uterine bleeding, nosebleeds, and blood in the urine. They are a diuretic and offer support to the kidney detoxification process.

Contraindications: Avoid nettles if you have severe kidney disease, are on dialysis, or have fluid retention due to congestive heart failure. Nettles may interfere with blood anticoagulant medication.

Linden Flowers *Tilia* spp.

There is a linden tree in Prospect Park, in Brooklyn, not too far from my home, where I take my apprentices when we do plant-identification walks. Every time I gather them under this specific linden tree, we have a spiritual experience. The feeling of safety and of being home and held is undeniable. Historically, branches of linden are hung over doorways for protection.

A benevolent Jupiter plant, Linden is called the tree of immortality and said to grant its user a long, sweet life. I have used linden after heartbreaks to restore my heart's resilience and open up again to joy. Use the leaves to call in love and magical dreams.

Linden (or Tilia, as it is known in other cultures) is an excellent circulatory nervine. It relieves nervous tension and spasms, and it is useful for treating high blood pressure, body pain from stress, heart palpitations, varicose veins, migraines, colds, fever, and flu.

Contraindications: Avoid long-term use or if the user is allergic to its pollen.

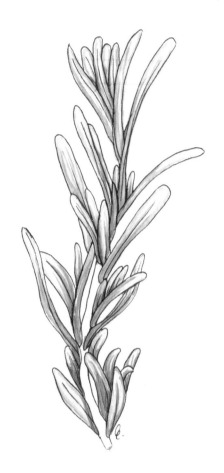

Rosemary *Salvia rosmarinus*

Rosemary has a diversity of uses as plant medicine. I use rosemary multiple times a week, and it is one of my favorite plants to use for protection. I use it in a protection spray and bath I make for Sacred Botanica, our spiritual shop where we focus on using plants for energetic purposes. Recently I have used it in a footbath and as face steam.

Rosemary/Romero is found in most households and is popular for cooking and seasoning our food. Connecting to its medicinal uses is as easy as asking people how their ancestors use this herb. When I teach rosemary, I learn from others how to further my use of this beautiful plant.

Plant of the Sun and Fire, rosemary brightens the mind and eases depression. Use this plant to rejuvenate and uplift the spirit when grieving through a loss. Rosemary invigorates the body and tones the nervous system. Use it to treat poor peripheral circulation, causing cold hands and feet. As a circulatory tonic, it aids memory loss and tension headaches. Use externally as a skin wash for wrinkles, bruises, and to strengthen capillaries. Make it into an herbal oil to rub into varicose veins and cellulite.

Contraindications: During pregnancy, avoid in large doses. Use it only as a seasoning for your food.

Heart Heal Syrup

Syrups are a great way to bring sweetness and tenderness to a broken heart or grieving heart. I have used this recipe to give my community a gift anytime there is a need to heal the heart. This recipe uses dried herbs, but freshly harvested herbs are also delicious. If using fresh plants, double the measurements for the herbs.

2 tablespoons (18 g) dried hawthorn berries

2 tablespoons (18 g) dried rose hips

2 tablespoons (18 g) dried raspberries

1 tablespoon (6 g) dried gingerroot

1 cup (340 g) organic honey

1 cup (235 ml) brandy

1 tablespoon (15 ml) edible rosewater

Yield: 1 quart (1 L)

Add the hawthorn berries, rose hips, raspberries, and gingerroot to a medium-size pot with 4 cups (940 ml) water. Simmer on the stove for 30 to 45 minutes.

Remove the decoction from the stove and strain it into a clean measuring cup. Stir the honey into the decoction until the honey blends. Add the brandy to the mixture and stir well.

Pour the syrup into a clean glass jar. Add the rosewater, shake well, cover, and label. This syrup can be taken by the tablespoon 3 times a day.

Store the unused syrup in the refrigerator. Discard after 45 days or when you see mold.

4th Chakra Heart Oil

Whenever I hear of a broken heart, I recommend anointing with a heart oil to heal. I have used rose essential oil in this way with my customers for many years in my apothecary. I like to use this recipe because it draws in other healing herbs' strength to move any stagnation and grief and speed heart healing. The practice of anointing the heart itself is healing, as it encourages self-touch.

This recipe is beneficial when doing the work of remembering our ancestral resilience and healing generational trauma. The 4th Chakra Heart Oil is also great for self-love and compassion work, grief, and loss, particularly after heartbreaks. It helps us get back in touch with a hardened or closed-off heart.

Use dried plant material when making herbal oils to prevent molding and bacteria.

¼ cup (8 g) dried roses

1 tablespoon (3 g) dried rosemary

1 teaspoon crushed cinnamon stick

1 teaspoon dried gingerroot

¾ cup (175 ml) sunflower or olive oil

Rose essential oil

Yield: 6 ounces (170 g)

Add the roses, rosemary, cinnamon, and gingerroot to a completely dry wide-mouth mason jar. Cover the plant material with the sunflower oil. Label your jar and set it in your sunniest window for 4 to 6 weeks.

After that time, using a cheesecloth or a fine-mesh strainer, strain off the plant material. Retain the oil, and discard the plants, or add it to a bath or footbath. Place 60 to 100 drops of the oil into a 6-ounce (170 ml) bottle. Add drops of the rose essential oil to your liking. Shake well and label your bottle. When preserved with essential oil, the shelf life of this oil is 6 months. Please store in a cool, dry place outside of direct sunlight.

Use as much oil as you need to anoint your heart. This oil is a good breast/chest massage oil. Our breast/chest sits right over our hearts and connects to any emotions held there.

Stress-Free Tea

This tea recipe is a preventative to stressors, and it is a great tea to relax the nerves and calm the heart when needed. It can be taken at bedtime, although the herbs do not have strong sleep-inducing properties. I drink this tea throughout the day while working on stressful deadlines or needing to center myself when dealing with a heavy workload. It is a beneficial formula when healing high blood pressure.

2 tablespoons (4 g) dried linden flowers

1 tablespoon (2 g) dried rose

1 tablespoon (2 g) dried hawthorn leaves and flowers

1 tablespoon (3 g) dried chamomile flowers

1 tablespoon (3 g) dried rosemary

Honey (optional)

Yield: 4 cups (940 ml)

Place all the ingredients in a 1-quart (1L) wide-mouth mason jar. Pour boiling water over the herbs and fill the jar. Let the herbs infuse for at least 25 minutes, then strain off the plant material. Retain the tea, and discard the plants, or add it to a bath or footbath. If you desire, sweeten your tea with honey and enjoy it throughout your day. When stored in the fridge, herbal tea can last for 2 days.

Ancestral Practice: Finding the Heart and Hawthorn: A Walking Meditation

For many of us who find it challenging to meditate, walking meditation is best. I like to purposefully interrupt my day and call myself back into my body by taking a walk in the park. Take the time to dedicate an afternoon when the weather is supportive for this meditation. You might need a map of the park or city blocks you plan on walking, or you may want to wander. Give yourself plenty of time to move without having to do the next task.

Take a blanket, a pen or pencil, and a journal to draw or write your thoughts in. Bring an offering for hawthorn and the Spirit of Oggun, such as rum, tobacco, a song, or a stone. You can support this practice by taking some Stress-Free Tea (page 29) with you to drink before and after the meditation.

Meditation: Finding Your Heart and Hawthorn

Begin by walking through your community looking for a hawthorn tree. When you come upon the tree, approach it with reverence. Stand under the tree and make your offering to the tree. Place it close to the tree's roots.

Lay out your blanket and lie or sit still comfortably. Feel the earth under you, holding you in safety, and thank her. Call in protection from Spirit, Oggun, the orisha of courage, your ancestors, and your guides.

When you are ready, picture yourself walking downstairs into your heart. Take each step with intention. See how far you get without arising too much anxiety. If so, challenge yourself for one more step and commit to trying again. Note when you stopped and what if any feelings, memories, and remembrances came up for you. If you need to stop, slowly open your eyes and praise yourself for making it as far as you did. Lie still in meditation until you are ready to come out of the practice.

If you made it down the stairs into your heart, take a look around: What do you see? Notice light, soft places and dark, closed, untouched, or unexplored places. Remember. Spend some time there and praise your heart for its strength, resilience, and joy.

Ask yourself: What do you want to add to what you see? What do you want to leave there, such as a rose quartz in a corner, a hawthorn berry, or a song reminding you of how courageous you are? Do you want to add a comfortable space for when you return? Leave something there that will connect you back when you reenter.

When finished, walk slowly up the stairs, and open your eyes. Lay still, basking in your meditation. When ready, journal your experience. Be compassionate with yourself and commit to returning to this particular tree and this practice. Thank the tree and Spirit, Oggun, ancestors, and guides for keeping your heart protected. Spend however long you need there to commune with the essence of hawthorn.

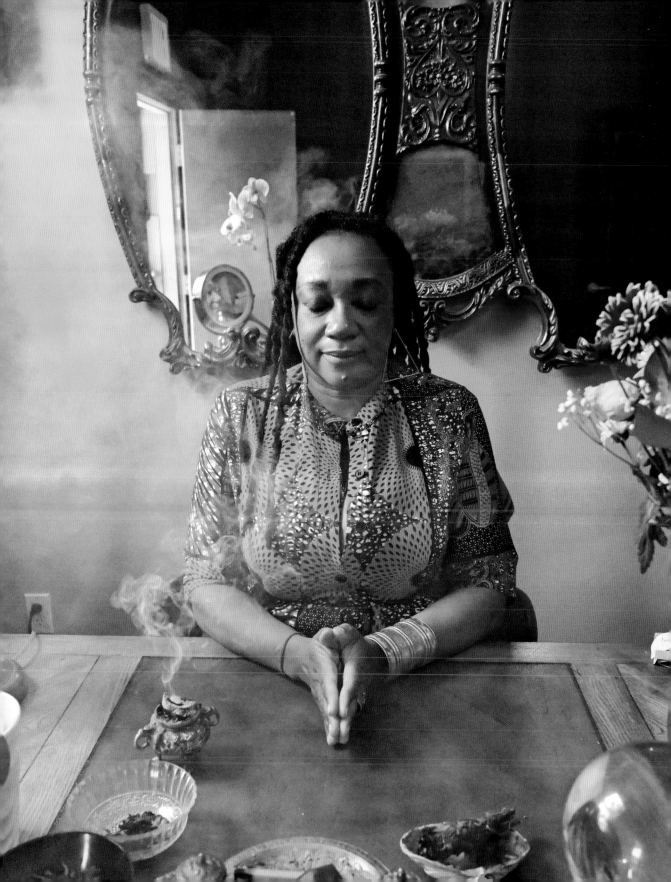

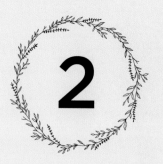

2

Being Present to Grief
RESPIRATORY HEALTH

———

Our bodies store away unexpressed grief and sadness in our lungs. Grief is persistent: Though we may not communicate it, it continues to exist, held in our bodies. Unprocessed familial grief does not disappear; it travels through the generations.

Respiratory illnesses are often an indicator of lineages of sorrow and grief buried in the lungs. I have had people come to the apothecary and say, "My family has had a cough they can't get rid of, my mother has a cough, my grandmother has a cough." With guidance, they trace back through the generations and notice that there is deep unexpressed grief that no one is addressing. This grief, such as a loss we have not grieved through, now develops into lung problems such as chronic bronchitis, asthma, or other lung issues.

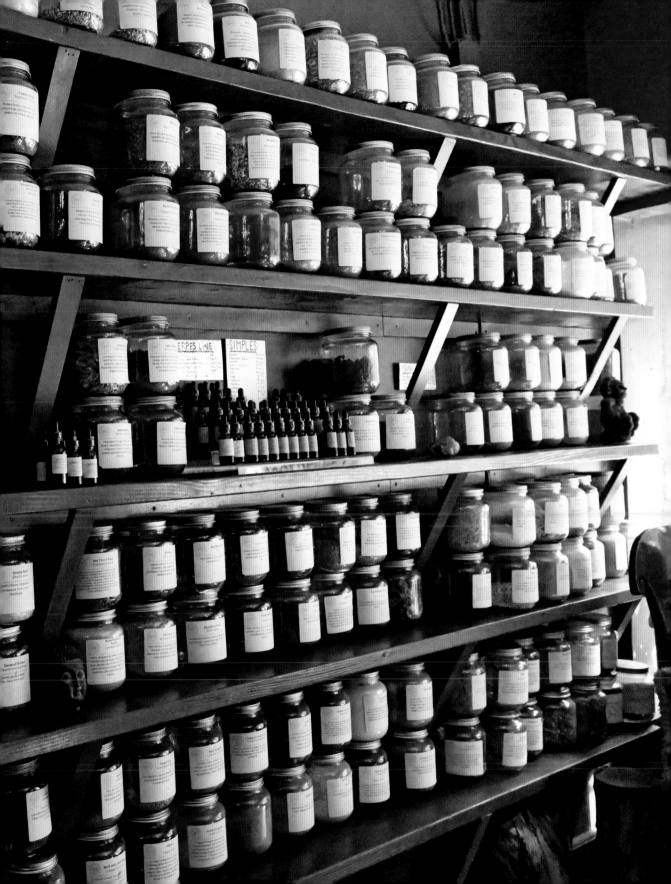

It is no wonder that descendants of enslaved people with ancestral trauma and grief pass lung disease from one generation to the next. Many families have a legacy of secrecy and silence, not wanting to talk about the sadness. I say to families who have shrouded themselves in silence that hereditary issues are not going anywhere until they are brought to light and exposed for healing.

Healing needs truth. Until the truth comes, healing will not happen. There is no true healing without accountability and integrity. Witness the effect of the family's loss and grieve it together, instead of pushing it down, storing it in our cells, and passing it on.

The Spirit of the Respiratory System

The respiratory system is the energy of Mercury. The orisha Elegba/Eshu—the messenger to the Gods—holds the power of communication. We must go through Elegba/Eshu for all our requests to the Divine. This domain extends to our lungs, throat, hands, speech, and hearing.

As the orisha at the crossroads, Elegba/Eshu opens doors for us to walk through, offering us a new path each time we breathe and use our voice. Each breath is a prayer and creates a new opportunity to express ourselves, trusting in the power of our expression to transform our lives.

A decisive voice is a messenger that clears the way for our growth and development. Open communication—which includes deep listening—can remove any obstacles we might encounter on this path. Remember: There is no protection when we are indecisive or allow doubt and fear to impede the next step forward. It is there that we meet with the "Devil," who is often associated with Eshu.

Breath and Voice

Breath and voice are deeply connected. Notice how we speak when we are struggling for breath versus being seated in our breath. We live in a world dominated by fear. Collectively we are all holding our breath. We have heard the expressions waiting to exhale, holding our breath, waiting for that other shoe to drop. The fear associated with releasing and holding on creates panic in our bodies. Often when something impacts us intensely, the first thing we lose is our breath. Bad news can knock the wind out of us, taking our breath and voice away.

Fear shows up in the breath when we hold on tight and do not trust enough to let go. Our breath is an exchange; as we breathe, our lungs rapidly exchange life-giving oxygen with carbon dioxide. The way we communicate is our exchange with the world. It is the way we give and receive. The giving is our out-breath, and we receive through our in-breath.

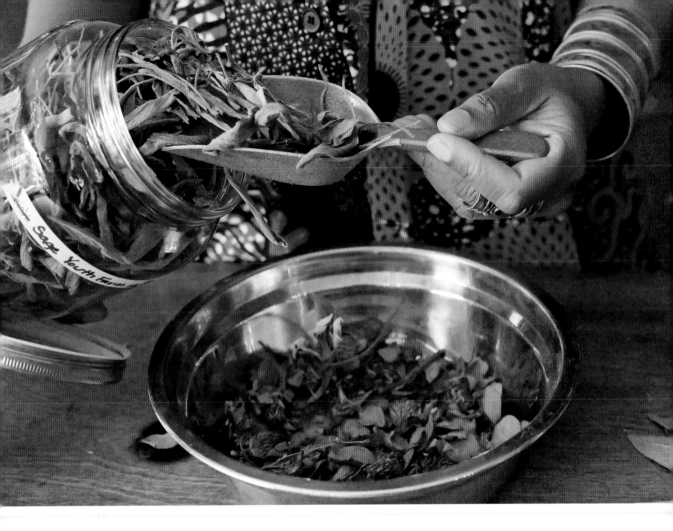

Many of us are great givers and not receivers. We continuously give without keeping anything for ourselves, which reflects in our breath. But some of us are receivers and not givers. We hold the out-breath, refusing to give because we sense fear, scarcity, and feelings of not being enough. Ultimately breathing is about trust.

Over my years of teaching, people have shared that they started having respiratory issues after a traumatic life event. Many people come into the apothecary and say, "I have always had this breathing problem." My question to them is, when did this happen? We trace it back to their childhood when their voice was not heard or they did not speak up due to fear. As your voice disappears, so does your breath, and you will likely face lung challenges.

Our breath signifies the power of expression in our own lives, while existing in interdependent relationships. The breath reflects the separation from our mother, demonstrating independence. Asthma can be related to codependency with the mother, never having the space to feel independent, or pushed into early autonomy. Lung issues can demonstrate the weight of having to shoulder being a parent and parenting your parent(s).

Any of our issues with our throat connect to the way we express ourselves. Censored and repressed speech in our childhood homes causes many children to stutter and find a lack of safety in their expression. We also see this inability to express in intimate relationships. Many smokers smoke to have an outward expression, the exchange of the out-breath. I often ask those who have come to me for help with smoking, where did you lose your voice?

As the breast sits on top of your lungs, breast cancer can also be related to grief, unexpressed creativity, and repression from living our most creative lives with a voice.

The Respiratory System

Each minute we breathe in and out, unconsciously, between ten and fifteen times. That's around 25,000 times a day! With each breath, our body extracts the oxygen it needs and discharges the blood's waste carbon dioxide.

Air enters through the nasal cavity, passes through the larynx and trachea/windpipe, enters the lungs, and moves into the bronchi and alveoli. The lungs are 10 percent tissue and 90 percent air. Their primary function is to exchange oxygen with carbon dioxide rapidly. One-third of the air we breathe is oxygen; the rest is nitrogen, carbon dioxide, bacteria, viruses, tobacco smoke, car exhaust, and other pollutants.

Through the blood, the cells of our body get supplied with oxygen. The circulatory system and the respiratory system bear most of this responsibility. The medulla oblongata controls this process in the brain, sending messages back and forth to regulate breathing.

If respiratory problems inhibit the exchange of gases in the lungs, body health can decline. Any problems with breathing affect organs and systems, and the reverse is also true: Any issues we have with other body systems (e.g., the circulatory system) can affect our breathing. When one system does not function correctly, the other becomes overtaxed. Our lungs are an eliminative organ and affect the function of other eliminative organs: our colon, skin, liver, and kidneys.

Notice Your Breath

Our breathing is unconscious, and our lungs function independently without us having to decide to breathe. Even though breathing is an unconscious function, choose conscious breathing by stopping and paying attention to your breath. Realize how your breath signals all the functions throughout the entire body.

You can enhance the health of the whole body by practicing conscious breathing. The entire day can pass, and we may never breathe below our diaphragm. The ability to sit for a few moments each day and breathe deeply is incredibly healing. Make it a regular practice to take a moment to center yourself and exchange breath. Take a full breath deep into the stomach, from below the diaphragm, and feel it into your belly. Notice how different that feels.

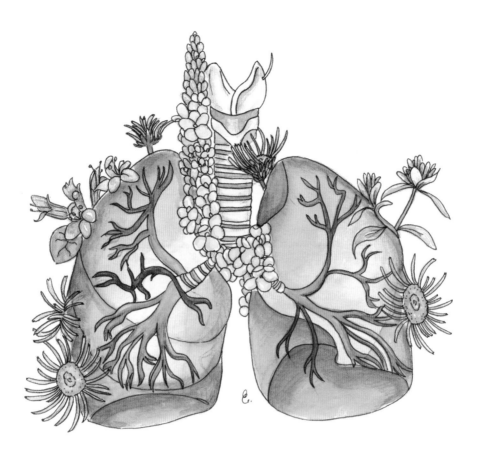

Plants for the Respiratory System

The herbs for the respiratory system allow us to express old grief and hurt. They help us heal from ancestral trauma that affects our voice. These plants heal the silence and lack of mourning that happens when we cannot express our sorrow. They reach into places where we may have become stagnated and usher in relief. They prepare us to have difficult conversations by softening and opening the heart and hearing to encourage deep listening and empathy.

Respiratory issues are significant in these times, and environmental factors contribute to many of them. Disasters and poor air quality in the industrial cities we call home negatively affect the air we breathe. This air affects all the organs in our bodies. Use these plants to reduce the harm and include them in your routine to maintain good respiratory health.

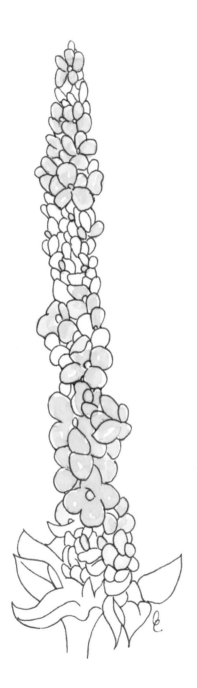

MULLEIN

Mullein heals by creating mental space. It opens up a congested and closed-off mind and heart, and it softens our approach to allow for reconnection and improved communication. This plant's healing can help someone who is not ready to deal with pain or grief, someone in denial and refusing to connect to the real issue.

The flowers of mullein are perfect for improving listening, and they foster courageous and empathetic conversations. They help you get in touch with your inner self, your authentic and genuine voice.

Common Name: Mullein

Latin Name: *Verbascum thapsus*

Other Names: Bunny Ears, Jacob's Staff, Flannel Flower, Velvet Leaf, Aaron's Rod, Candlewick Plant

Taxonomy: Scrophulariaceae

Botanical Description: Mullein has biannual yellow flowers that grow on a stalk. The big, soft leaves are covered in small hairs.

Native Habitat: West Europe and Asia; naturalized in North America

Wildcrafting and Cultivation: Harvest leaves before or after the plant flowers. The plant will flower in its second year. Grow by seed in well-drained soil in direct sunlight.

Parts Used: Leaves, flowers

Planetary Influence/Correspondence:
Saturn, Fire, Yin

Energetic Quality: Bitter, astringent, sweet,
pungent, cool

Pharmacological Constituents: Mucilage;
flavonoids; saponins; essential oils; tannins; glyco-
side; complex carbohydrates; plant sterols; sugars

Ethnobotanical/Historical Use: Flower
stalks were dipped in lard and used as torches.
Farmers gave mullein to cattle to prevent them
from coughing. Indigenous Americans used
mullein for medicine and smoking. Quaker girls
rubbed the leaves on their cheeks to redden them,
so mullein earned the name "Quaker Rouge."

Actions/Properties: Antitussive; expectorant;
demulcent; diuretic; anti-inflammatory; antispasmodic; antituberculosis; nervine; vulnerary;
alterative; astringent; anodyne; antimicrobial;
antioxidant; cancer preventative; great children's
remedy

Indications: *Leaf:* Lung and bronchial issues;
spasmodic coughs; emphysema; bronchitis with
a hard and painful cough; sore throat; tuberculosis; nervousness; insomnia *Flower:* Ear infections;
laryngitis; pharyngitis; lymphatic congestion;
urinary tract infection; eczema of the ear

Contraindications: The seeds of mullein are
toxic. Avoid mullein if you have "high Vata" conditions (people who are light and airy). Use only
externally with cancer because it moves lymph.

Methods of Preparation and Dosage

Infusion: Use 1 tablespoon (15 ml) to 1 cup (235
ml) boiling water. Steep for 20 to 25 and use 3
times a day. Strain it well because the small hairs
on the leaves can irritate the throat.

Tincture: Use 15 to 30 drops of the tincture 3
times a day.

External Applications: Smoke mullein leaves
for lung issues such as bronchitis and asthma.
Use mullein flowers oil for ear infections and
eczema of the ear: add 5 to 10 drops of warm
oil into the ear cavity. Use a strong tea of mullein
for herpes breakouts or as a compress for acne,
bruises, earache, eczema, or mastitis: add ¼ cup
(60 ml) to 1 cup (235 ml) boiling water, let sit for
at least 2 hours, and use as a wound wash.

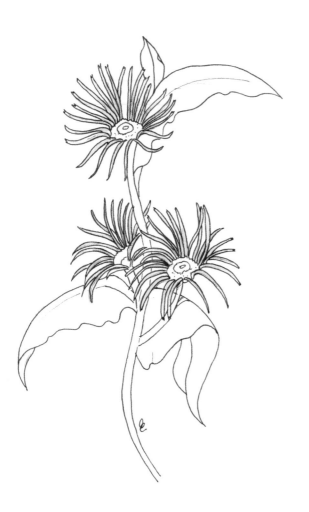

ELECAMPANE

Elecampane provides shelter, expression, and comfort in times of profound grief. This plant flourished in our box outside Sacred Vibes Apothecary. The leaves were large, and it was flowering; it looked like the princess of plants on the block. We noticed two pigeons near the plant; they stayed there together for a week, and one day they were gone. That evening I was pointing out to my associate how beautiful this plant was. I looked under the leaf, and one pigeon was dead there. We recognized that the pigeon chose to die under the elecampane leaf and the other pigeon stood by in vigil, offering comfort and companionship. The same thing happened the second summer that plant was with us. These birds instinctively knew elecampane's power.

Use elecampane's medicine to heal the loss of displacement and migration, for those grieving their home and homeland's loss. It is beautiful medicine for connecting with unexpressed sadness. It supports healing from generational trauma by bringing grief to the surface. Elecampane's energy is warm, yang, and ruled by Mercury and Air. It removes stagnation and gives us the words to express so we may get to the other side of grieving.

Common Name: Elecampane

Latin Name: *Inula helenium*

Other Names: Scabwort, Elfdock, Horseheal, Yellow Starwort

Taxonomy: Asteraceae

Botanical Description: Elecampane is 3 to 6 feet (1 to 2 m) tall with thick branches, large ovate leaves, and bright yellow flower heads.

Native Habitat: Europe; roadsides of eastern and central United States and Canada

Wildcrafting and Cultivation: Collect the root when the plant is dormant. This plant is easy to grow by seed or with a piece of root. It needs two years to grow before harvesting the root.

Parts Used: Roots

Planetary Influence/Correspondence: Sun, Mercury, Air

Energetic Quality: Aromatic, bitter, pungent, yang

Pharmacological Constituents: Inula; helenin; polysaccharides

Ethnobotanical/Historical Use: Called "horseheal" because of its use to treat lung disorders in horses. Called "scabwort" because it was used to heal scabs on sheep. In Rome the roots were candied and eaten for digestive issues and when overeating. Candied elecampane root was still sold up to fifty years ago in London. Legend has it that when Helen of Troy was torn away from her home, her tears fell, and elecampane grew in the places where they fell.

Actions/Properties: Richest source of inulin (a nutrient-dense starch); tonic; diaphoretic; expectorant; alterative; antiseptic; astringent; gentle stimulant; antitussive; carminative; hepatic; antimicrobial; bronchodilator; lung tonic

Indications: Coughs and shortness of breath; old bronchial and sinus conditions; all lung complaints; bronchitis; chest infections with stiffness; asthma; emphysema; whooping cough; tuberculosis; flu; tonsillitis; postnasal drip; rattling cough; damp lung conditions; digestive issues

Contraindications: Do not use during pregnancy, the early stages of nursing, or in the presence of ulcers or diarrhea.

Methods of Preparation and Dosage

Decoction: Simmer 1 teaspoon in 2 cups (475 ml) water for 20 to 25 minutes. Drink ¼ cup (60 ml) up to 3 times a day.

Tincture: Use 1 dropper or 30 drops of tincture 3 times a day for chronic issues.

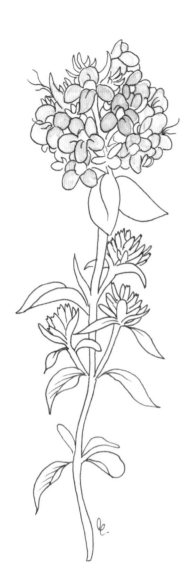

THYME

Spiritually thyme is associated with the Dead, as it supports release and letting go. It helps us develop a better relationship with time, connects us to our breath, and keeps us in the present. It is excellent for the fear associated with the out-breath release, causing tension and spasms in the lungs. It is protective and used to relieve and prevent nightmares.

Thyme also facilitates time traveling. It is associated with jumping linear time lines in the space-time continuum, which is especially useful for generational healing. Use the incense and in spells to draw ancestral Spirits closer and to speed healing.

Thyme is accessible and easy to grow, and most of us have used thyme in our food. In Caribbean households, there is no cooking without thyme. One of my favorite uses of thyme is in a honey taken to prevent and treat colds and flu. It is an excellent remedy for a sore throat.

Common Name: Thyme

Latin Name: *Thymus vulgaris*

Other Names: Common Thyme, Garden Thyme

Taxonomy: Lamiaceae

Botanical Description: Thyme is a small shrub with linear to elliptic leaves. Some varieties spread, and some are upright. The plant has small white to light purple flowers.

Native Habitat: Western Mediterranean to southern Italy; Spain; Siberia; naturalized everywhere

Wildcrafting and Cultivation: Sow seeds in January. Thyme likes full sun; protect its leaves in summer.

Parts Used: Leaves, flowering tops, essential oil

Planetary Influence/Correspondence: Venus, Water

Energetic Quality: Spicy, pungent, warm

Pharmacological Constituents: Volatile oils; bitter principle; tannins; flavonoids; acids; vitamins B, C, and D

Ethnobotanical/Historical Use: Medicinal use of thyme dates to 3000 BCE. It was a symbol of courage to the Greeks. It is used as a temple incense and burned as purification and as a sacrifice to God. It was used to drive away insects and infections, ease melancholy, and ward off negativity and nightmares. Thyme symbolized death in certain cultures.

Actions/Properties: Carminative; antiseptic; expectorant; antitussive; antimicrobial; antibacterial; astringent; antifungal; antiparasitic; emmenagogue; aromatic; diaphoretic; immune enhancer

Indications: Coughs, colds, and flu; indigestion; ringworm; athlete's foot; tooth decay; gum infections; headaches; delayed menses

Contraindications: Do not use as medicine during pregnancy; use only to season food.

Methods of Preparation and Dosage

Infusion: Use 1 tablespoon (15 ml) to 1 cup (235 ml) water. Steep for 20 to 25 minutes, and drink hot. Drink 1 cup (235 ml) up to 3 times a day.

Tincture: Use 15 to 30 drops of tincture 3 times a day.

External Use: Use thyme tea as a wash or footbath for athlete's foot.

ADDITIONAL PLANTS

Osha *Ligusticum porteri*

I was introduced to osha while living in Arizona, where I was given the root by a friend whose ancestors were native to this land. When I first tasted osha, I knew this was strong medicine. I remember the distinctive taste and the tingling feeling in my mouth. I immediately felt connected to the plant and felt its draw into a relationship. This plant lets you know if it wants to be your ally; take the time to listen carefully. Thyme is an excellent substitute for osha's medicine, but I have included osha here because, over the years, it has been a close ally and friend to me.

Osha, or Bear Medicine, as named by Americas' indigenous peoples, is a warrior plant guided by Mars and Fire. It grows on mountains up 7,500 feet (2,300 m) in altitude, and because of its habitat, it knows how to utilize oxygen. Osha oxygenates our bodies, adding up to 10 to 15 percent more usable oxygen.

Osha is a protective guide in the dreamworld, and I still remember all of my dreams while walking osha. (See page 30 to learn more about walking with a plant.) Osha enhances psychic abilities and intuition, and it deepens your communication with the Spirit world. It is an endangered plant and ancestral medicine, and it is revered and considered sacred by indigenous peoples of this land. If called to walk with this plant, carry it in a red cloth. (Red is the color of power and sacredness; plants such as osha and comfrey are traditionally carried in a red cloth.)

Osha's energy is direct and powerful, and it should only be used for acute conditions. A tincture of osha is best. The root of the plant is excellent for bacterial and viral infections. I have used it successfully for sinus and lung infections, bronchitis, sore throat, fever, cough, and colds. It is a strong diaphoretic and is best taken at the onset of symptoms, as it opens the sweat glands so you can release toxins through the skin.

Contraindications: Do not use during pregnancy and breast/chest feeding. Make a positive identification of this plant before harvesting. Use only when needed, as this plant is endangered.

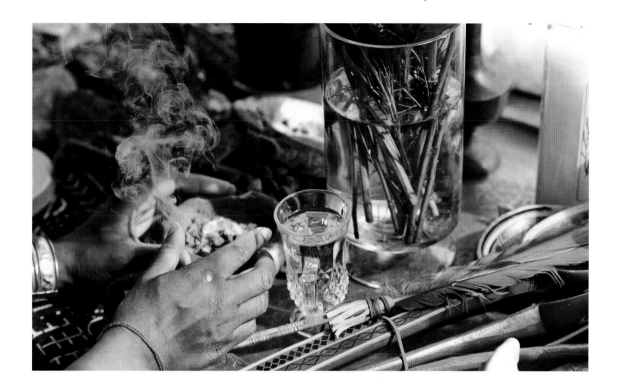

Oregano *Origanum* spp.

Oregano, known as Joy of the Mountain, is a plant guided by Mercury and Air, Eshu/Elegba energy. It is useful for breathwork that strengthens the breath and creates an openness to communication with lightness and joy. It is protective against those who interfere and are troublesome in their energy. I often use it to keep joyless people at bay. Use oregano to add intensity to love and prosperity spells.

Like thyme, oregano is accessible medicine. It is a common garden plant that most people have a relationship with as seasoning for food. One of my favorite ways to use this plant, other than to cook with it, is in respiratory steams to clear sinuses, relieving sinus pressure and headaches. Oregano is drying and warming in energy and is anti-inflammatory and antiseptic. It is useful for asthma, bronchitis, cough, fever, and flu.

Contraindications: Avoid large doses during pregnancy, but it is safe to use as a seasoning.

Clear Voice Smoke Blend

Over the years one best-seller at Sacred Vibes Apothecary is our smoke blends. They are a great way to allow the release of breath and open up the lungs using supportive lung plants. Many of my customers substitute an herbal smoking blend to lessen their dependence on cigarettes and heal the lungs after years of damage. I use smoke blends to relax, encourage dreams, for meditation, and for visions. Use smoke blends moderately, as any regular smoking can affect lung health.

This blend I am sharing with you helps open the throat to encourage clear communication with others and the Spirit world.

1 tablespoon (3 g) dried mullein leaves

1 tablespoon (3 g) dried thyme leaves

1 tablespoon (3 g) dried damiana leaves

1 teaspoon dried peppermint leaves

1 teaspoon dried red raspberry leaves

Yield: 2.5 ounces (70 g)

Combine all of the plant materials in a mortar or small bowl. Break them down using your pestle, a plant grinder, or your hands. When broken down, using your hands, mix the plants well in a clean bowl. Add a sprinkle of water to moisten the herbs. Using rolling papers, roll plants into an herbal cigarette or smoke them in a pipe.

Thyme and Ginger Honey

This honey is an easy recipe I have used to introduce people to the simplicity of healing with herbs. I ask them to use what they have in their homes to create medicine. I often substitute the thyme or ginger with onion and garlic. Have fun and include children in this preparation, as it is one medicine I find useful for them during cold and flu season. I prefer to make this recipe with fresh plants and use the no-heat method of preparation. Use half as much if you prefer to use dried.

3 sprigs fresh thyme

4 slices fresh ginger
(a 1-inch [2.5 cm] piece)

4 ounces (120 g) organic liquid honey

Yield: 4 ounces (120 g)

Place the thyme and ginger slices in a clean wide-mouth mason jar. Cover the plant material entirely with the honey. Shake the jar well and place it on a sunny windowsill, letting the plants infuse for 4 to 6 weeks in the honey. Turn the jar over each time you pass by.

After at least 4 weeks, strain out the plant material using a fine-mesh sieve. Don't discard the plants; add them to a tea or sweeten up a lemonade.

Store the infused honey in a clean glass jar and use by the tablespoons. I recommend taking 1 tablespoon (20 g) of the honey each day as a preventative and treatment for a cold, flu, or sore throat.

Breathe Easy Steam

With the COVID-19 pandemic, many people who never used herbal medicines began to seek out and use plants for respiratory steaming. It is an easy and effective way to improve respiratory health. Steaming decongests nasal passages and opens up bronchial passages for deeper breathing. Using plants that are antimicrobial and antibacterial prevents and treats infections in the upper respiratory tract.

Steams are great medicine to use with children, as they bring an essence of play while tenting the head and allowing the steam to work. I have used this steam since my children were young. Use fresh or dried plants.

1 tablespoon (3 g) dried eucalyptus leaves

1 tablespoon (3 g) dried peppermint leaves

1 tablespoon (3 g) dried thyme leaves

1 tablespoon (3 g) dried oregano leaves

Yield: 1 steam

Mix all the plants in a large glass bowl. Find a comfortable seat and pour 3 to 4 cups (705 to 940 ml) boiling water over the plants. Lean over the bowl and tent your head with a towel, preventing the steam from escaping. Bend your head over the bowl for at least 10 minutes, then take a break, and, if desired, return to steaming. You may need to add additional hot water to create more steam.

When done, you can add more hot water and use it in a bath, footbath, or vaginal steam (see page 114) before discarding the plant material.

Ancestral Practice: Ritual Smoking: A Breath Practice

This practice utilizes an herbal smoking blend. Use the one on page 46 or choose one you like. I generally sit in front of my altar at home when engaging in my ritual smoking practice. If this doesn't work for you, find a safe and comfortable space to sit.

Roll an herbal cigarette—or some use a cigar to honor Eshu/Elegba for this practice. Within Ifá and other traditional religious practices and ceremonies, smoke is used to cleanse or to send messages on. Elegba, being the messenger, is honored by cigars. I have found that designating and consecrating a favorite pipe with prayer adds a special reverence to this practice.

Ritual smoking is an ancient practice in many cultures and is used like prayer to communicate with Spirit and the ancestors. The smoke is our words, our breath, and our intention sent out into the Universe. I have found this smoking ritual to be incredibly healing, as it uses breathwork to connect us to unhealed grief and trauma held in our bodies. Traumatic birth experiences, childhood trauma, and ancestral trauma all affect our breath. Using the breath, breathe deeply into your body, and see where these experiences are held and release them.

Ritual Smoking

Begin this practice by honoring the directions, as our indigenous family taught us: Start with the East and ask the gatekeeper to open the way for newness and inspiration. Face the South, and thank your Spirit, guides, and ancestors for the fire, the spark of life, and joy present in your heart. Next turn to the West and thank the grandmothers, the waters for their nourishing, generous, and cleansing spirit we take in each day. Turn to the North and thank the Spirit of the Ancestors for accompanying you always and showing up for you in dreamtime. Lift your hands and thank our Divine Father for all the blessings that come from the Sky. Touch the floor and thank our Mother Earth for feeding us, giving us a home, and all the gifts that come from the soil. Having called in this circle of protection and with reverence in your heart, have a seat.

Set your intention for this meeting with Spirit and your ancestors. What are your prayers for your body, your family and community, and the Universe? With your prayer in mind, light your pipe or herbal cigarette. Breathe in the plant's medicines deeply, noticing how it feels in your mouth and as it travels through your esophagus to your lungs. As you inhale, let that be the prayer for your body, and let your exhale be your offering and request from Spirit for your family and community.

When done, close the directions by turning to each direction and thanking the spirits, guides, and ancestors present. Send them on their journey back with your gratitude for prayers received and answered.

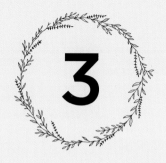

3

Following Your Gut
DIGESTIVE HEALTH

———

The digestive system is the middle way, the bridge across the gap between our roots, the ancestors, and our cosmic ascension, to the higher parts of the spiritual self, often called the gut-brain axis. This spiritual growth process occurs in the gut, where messages are received and sent to the brain, which initiates action.

Our instinct, awareness, and innate intelligence lie in our gut. I have heard many say, "I knew it! My gut told me!" The question then is, why didn't you listen? We are conditioned to listen to when our mind speaks, but what we feel is often considered secondary or ignored.

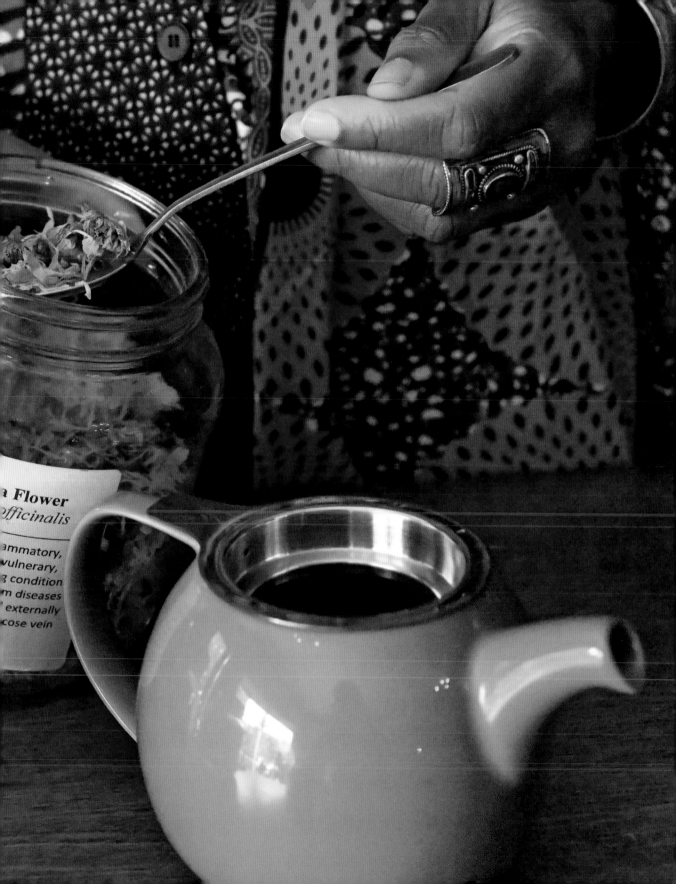

An unhealthy digestive system disconnects us from our instinct, feelings, and intuition. The ancients believed that our gut was our first brain. Everything we received was processed first by our digestive brain or the enteric nervous system, a mesh-like network of nerves that lives in the digestive tract. These nerves receive external messages and communicate them to the brain and body via the vagus nerve. Presently this nervous system is called the second brain because it operates independently outside the brain and spinal cord control.

In practice I recognize that the ancients were correct in calling our gut the first brain. We live in a hypermasculine, patriarchal culture that has programmed us to uphold the masculine thinking brain over the feminine feeling gut, giving the brain the ultimate authority over our actions. Nature upholds the feminine and honors that our intuition and feelings are sacred and precede our minds.

In our gut we sense feelings even before we can form a thought. Children and pets demonstrate what it means to function instinctively. As adults, we turn off that instinctive side. Refusing to trust our feelings, we lean into judgment and rationalization. It is a relearning to honor our intuition once again, to trust what we feel and not challenge that feeling with reason. Listening to your intuition is like building a muscle. The more we operate from a feeling-based place, the more we develop our intuitive powers.

Shutting off our egocentric brain and leaning into our intuition means developing deep listening, which sometimes requires a pause. Know that your intuition is your first voice and your thinking brain is always second. When making a decision, ask yourself: At this moment, how do I feel about this? Practice doing this several times a day. Focus not on what you think about this situation, but rather how you feel.

Our gut health and intuition are often affected by bodily trauma, emotional trauma, the trauma of poverty, and lack of access to healthy food sources. The foods we eat continue to deaden our stomach's brain. Without food sourced directly from nature, we lose our connection to our body's wisdom. Nature is in direct alignment with our listening. Everything in nature listens instinctively— animals, plants, soil, and water are all in direct communication with each other. The more we take natural foods into our body, the more our listening heightens.

The Art & Practice of SPIRITUAL HERBALISM

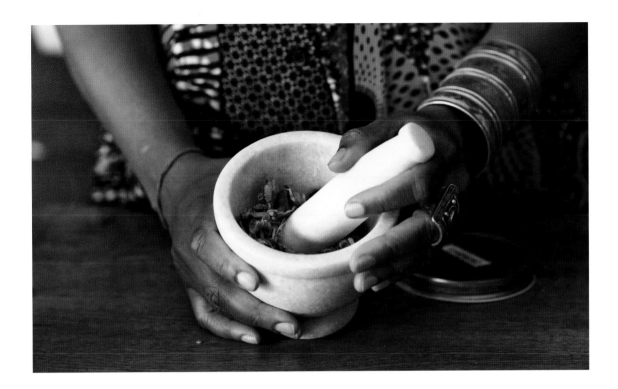

The Spirit of the Digestive System

Guided by the Moon, the digestive system is our emotional core linking us to our foundation and our family's core beliefs. Within our families, we develop what we believe spiritually and what we think about others, the world, and ourselves. We inherit beliefs around security, confidence, and relationships. We were taught all the things in our childhood that were inherently passed on to us, including beliefs around poverty, sexuality, food, scarcity, religion, and race. These core beliefs of the people who raised us influence our lives and health.

If you believe that you are not worthy, more than likely, your family has developed this belief over time. A child's worth and security come from their environment. Core beliefs, particularly the belief system of our mother lines—our mother, her mother, and her mother—are stored in the gut and influence our lives. Removing our familial programming demands that we look at beliefs that are now no longer our truth but remain held in our bellies. The digestive system's function is to digest, process, and eliminate. Digestive health means letting go of what no longer serves us.

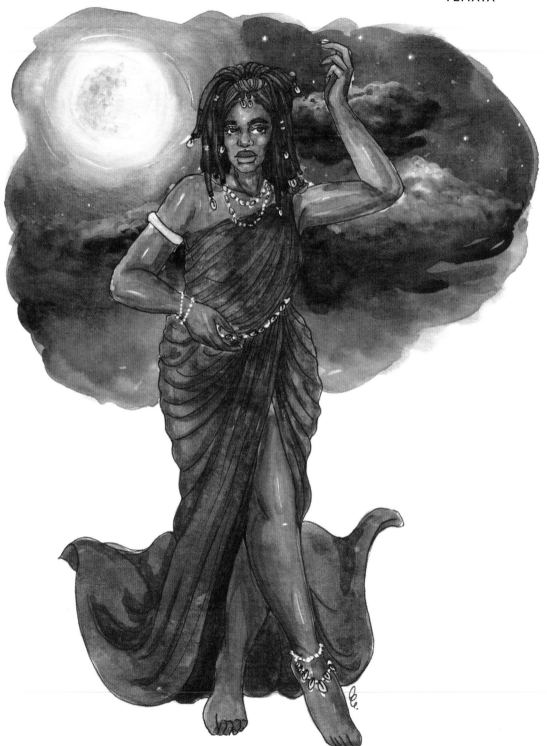

The Art & Practice of SPIRITUAL HERBALISM

Relationships and Mothers

The digestive system's guide is the energy of the ever-present mother, the Moon or Yemaya. Anything growing requires nurturing, and Yemaya mothers and nurtures her children. She symbolizes the relationship between mother and child. Our first and primary relationship is with our mothers, which began even before we were born. While in the uterus, we learned how to relate to our mothers and connected through the umbilical cord, right in the middle of our gut, passing messages back and forth. After birth, this learning continued as we watched our mothers teach us about relationships.

There is no way to avoid our mother's influence. The judgment attached to a mother-child relationship is palpable. Without healing, how the mother judges us then becomes how we judge ourselves and others. The parts of our mothers that make us uncomfortable are the parts that make us uncomfortable with ourselves.

The Moon reflects our mother's relationship with herself and the world. Not seeing ourselves as independent of our mothers, we worry we may become her. Our digestive system stores these feelings of worry, fear, judgment, rejection, abandonment, and unworthiness. How confident are we to step into the unknown in our power outside the shadow of mothers and know that we will thrive?

Our mothers' nurturing connects to our digestive system's health. Digestive dis-ease is the body's reminder to mother and nurture the self. Many of us did not receive a mother's care, compassion, and assurance. To heal ourselves means loving the child inside in all the ways we did not receive, including working to build our confidence and self-worth, being the voice of encouragement, and praising ourselves.

The Moon/Yemaya is the mother of oceans and guides the waters in our bodies, our emotions. Our moods and mental health are affected by our gut health. Our digestive health reflects any lack of emotional security. This feeling of emotional security also extends to our families and communities and all of our relationships.

The solar plexus in the gut represents the Sun, and the moon guides the digestive system. This Sun-Moon relationship highlights the relationship between Yemaya and Oshun, where our worth parallels our self-confidence. Oshun is the goddess of sensuality and the body. She represents what fullness can feel like when there is a well of nourishment springing from a well-nurtured source. Like the ocean, Yemaya feeds the sweet river and waterfalls, where Oshun lives. Confidence, beauty, power, and vulnerability come from compassionate care and nurture. Stories tell us that Oshun gets pregnant and gives birth, and Yemaya raises the children. These two orishas show us how care and nurturing prepare us for standing in our abundance and overflowing.

Mother's work is often the most challenging thing we have to do in this life. It requires compassion for ourselves primarily, knowing when we need to take a break and step away for self-care. Any attempts we make to heal ourselves heals the generation forward and generations backward. Even though they may not be at the table with you, they are benefiting.

The Digestive System

Over the years of teaching herbalism, I have strongly encouraged my students to know all their digestive system's parts and functions. Being able to express where any discomfort is coming from is essential. Our digestive health is a reflection and a mirror to the health of our entire body. It is one of the most important ways to understand how our bodies function and determine where and whether there is disease. Digestive problems are rampant, and most illnesses stem from them.

The appetite is a great place to be in touch with the health of the digestive system. What does a healthy appetite look like for you? Remember, normalcy is individual. You know your body best and can honor the need to adjust your food intake. Using our instincts, we can be aware of the natural messages our bodies send us and follow them to heal our digestive system.

Our ancestors knew that bitter foods promoted good digestion and included them in their daily diet. Many of our traditional foods are spicy and bitter. In our Western diet, we have replaced bitter with sweet. Most of our digestive enzymes that promote the absorption of nutrients come from bitter foods. Bitters produce digestive enzymes and bile in the liver, which is necessary for the breakdown of proteins and cleansing toxins from the body.

The digestive system comprises the mouth, salivary glands, esophagus, stomach, pancreas, small intestine, and large intestine. All of our digestive system parts are engaged in the breakdown and processing of what we take in. What we nourish ourselves with will show up in the health of the digestive system.

The health of our colon is primary to the health of our entire bodies. Common illnesses that stem from poor colon health include anxiety, asthma, candida, food cravings and fatigue, circulation issues, headaches, foggy brain, sluggish thinking, irritability, lack of libido, and skin issues such as eczema and acne.

Menstrual problems can occur when the womb feels pressure from an impacted colon. The colon sits right below the womb, and the womb expands to twice its size during menses. A full colon worsens cramping, spasms, and backache.

The colon is a muscular organ. If the muscle tone is poor, this could show up as chronic constipation. Fortunately herbs can help retrain our colon for peristalsis, the wave-like motion that causes movement. Strengthening the liver's function will support the colon.

The Art & Practice of SPIRITUAL HERBALISM

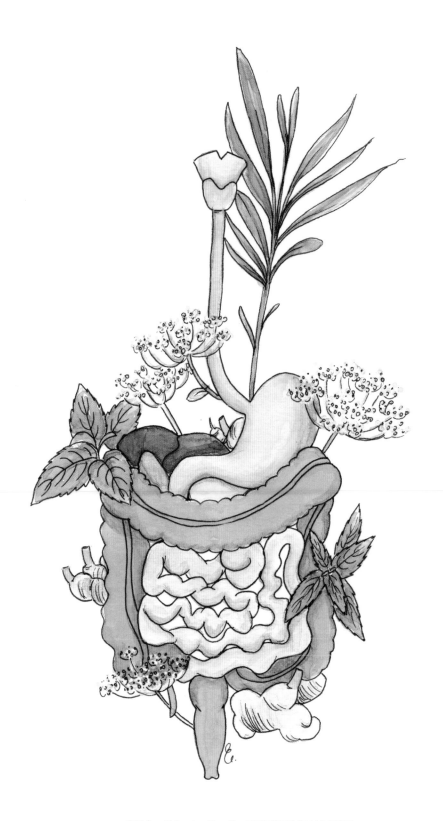

Decolonizing Our Relationship to Our Digestive System

We often have to examine our relationship with food to understand where a food addiction comes from and what has brought it forward. Beyond the food, we need to find what feeling it connects us to, and how far back it goes. Have we replaced nurturing with food? Are we punishing ourselves with food? It could be the memory of punishment attached to it, and we now choose to self-punish. Or it could be that the food brings with it a memory of the only times we felt nurtured.

Food recalls a memory and connects us to experiences. I had a client who came from Colombia as a child. She was eleven years old, fleeing the drug wars, and remembers her grandmother saying, "I can't go. The only thing I can give you is this bread recipe." But this client has an awful gluten allergy and could not stop eating bread. It was not the bread; it was the memory of what the bread connected her to, the memory of her grandmother, whom she would never see again, that she could not release. No one could tell her to stop eating bread until she was ready to release the memory of her grandmother.

I am an immigrant as well. At fourteen my family emigrated from Guyana. As displaced people, we connected our cultural foods to a sense of normalcy amid many changes. Our food from our home was part of our survival in this new place. It is a myth that cultural foods are inherently bad for our bodies. Many of our traditional foods are lifegiving, nutrientdense, and fuel our bodies for our daily work.

As people living in a new land, we have had to adjust our relationship to the land and food. Many of us grew our food; we lived in relationship to the land and ate what was seasonally available. Many become ill after having to adjust to packaged and processed foods and new digestive routines. One such illness I see rampant among displaced people is diabetes, which spiritually is the lack of joy and sweetness in our lives. We often seek to fill our loss of home, community, and family with sweetness from food, which is usually processed and filled with sugars, leading to diabetes and other illnesses.

Digestion and Routine

Decolonize your routine! Many cultures we come from honor mealtimes by establishing a nationwide lunch schedule where everyone eats at a particular time, rests, and then returns to work and is home by dinner. Our diets have become institutionalized, and we tend to eat based on what our work schedules dictate rather than what is best for our health. With the recent COVID-19 lockdown, many expressed how grateful they were to eat when they needed to.

A routine heals the digestive system. Digestive health isn't gained through the latest fad diet, nor does it function well when we eat our meals irregularly. Instead it follows the rhythms of the Earth and that which exists around us naturally.

Follow the Sun

Good digestion means allowing ourselves to feel and tune into the circadian rhythms, looking to the Sun as a guide.

- When rising, your breakfast, the first meal of the day, is a light meal in the morning. Bitter teas can help in the morning to break the fast we have been in all night.

- At midday, the Sun is at its highest peak; your digestive fire is now burning, and your body is ready to digest. It's time to have your largest meal. Your body is prepared for the large meal.

- In the evening as the Sun sets, we are ready to fast for the night, and our dinner should be lighter and easily digestible. Eating a large meal late leads to digestive distress.

- As we go into our overnight fast, the parasympathetic nervous system becomes more active to help the digestive process. The parasympathetic nervous system functions when we are at rest. If our bodies cannot find rest or we are not sleeping well at night, our digestive system cannot function well.

Think of ways you could add more of a routine in your life. Retrain your body to eat meals at the same time each day; this may mean taking food with you to stay on a schedule. I have asked many of my clients to keep a food journal, writing down everything they have eaten for the day and the time they ate. It is often eye-opening to see what they have been putting into their bodies and what they have neglected entirely. This practice is without judgment and done not to feel inadequate about our food choices. Instead it gives us a real sense of how we nourish ourselves each day. Try it!

Plants for the Digestive System

The plants recommended for the digestive system tap into the wisdom held in our enteric nervous system. They aid in digestion and are often warming; fiery plants bring heat to disconnected feelings and strengthen intuition. They warm up an individual who has cut themselves off from their emotions and heart, disconnected from their feelings. They are useful for grief, regret, trauma, and lack of forgiveness. These plants raise our vibration and encourage clarity and decision-making while honoring our deepest feelings.

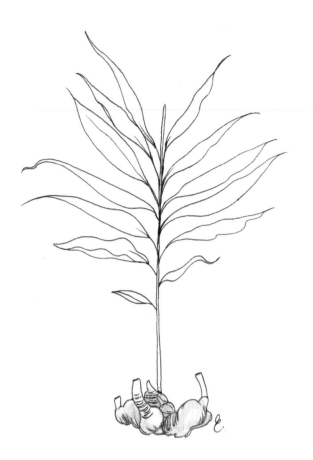

GINGER

This tropical, Mars/Oggun plant is ancestral medicine that has been around for thousands of years and was introduced to the West more than two thousand years ago. In the Caribbean, we joke that our grandmothers recommended ginger tea for every ailment under the Sun. Its energy is spicy, hot, aromatic, and dry. It's warming and brings life to the solar plexus, our place of power. It is the ideal third chakra medicine.

Ginger thaws frozen feelings. I call it medicine that breaks the emotional dam. It is excellent for those who need to let tears flow. I often use it with people who are ready to engage in forgiveness work with their families, as it inspires heartfelt communication.

Ginger is an accessible medicine, easily found in our communities at the corner bodega, vegetable market, and grocery store. It builds self-esteem and confidence. It's also excellent for rebuilding the body's fire and is useful for depression, including seasonal depression. Use it as a circulatory tonic and to nourish the giving and receiving nature of love.

Common Name: Ginger

Latin Name: *Zingiber officinale*

Other Names: African Ginger, Sheng Jiang (Chinese), Jengibre (Spanish)

Taxonomy: Zingiberaceae

Botanical Description: Gingerroot is a buff-colored, knobby, thick, scaly root that resembles hands. The plant has linear leaves alternately arranged on the stem, and it produces cone-shaped, pale yellow flowers.

The Art & Practice of SPIRITUAL HERBALISM

Native Habitat: Tropical plant; Asia; Jamaica; Haiti

Wildcrafting and Cultivation: Propagate by dividing rootstock. Sow in fertile soil, with lots of rain and warm, tropical conditions. Harvest when 6 to 10 months old and when the plant is not flowering.

Parts Used: Root, essential oil

Planetary Influence/Correspondence: Mars, Fire

Energetic Quality: Spicy, pungent, hot, dry

Pharmacological Constituents: Volatile oils; phenols; alkaloids; mucilage; nutrientdense; potassium; magnesium; sodium; vitamins A, B, and E; proteins; fats; antioxidants; calcium; capsaicin

Ethnobotanical/Historical Use: Ginger was cultivated in China and India and used for thousands of years. Romans added it to mulled wine for fertility and lust. The people of Arabia and Turkey used ginger as an aphrodisiac. The Chinese used it as a folk cure for vitiligo. English Puritans disliked it for its warming, aphrodisiac actions.

Actions/Properties: Analgesic; antacid; antiemetic; anti-inflammatory; antispasmodic; aperitive; aromatic; carminative; diaphoretic; diuretic; emmenagogue; nervine; rubefacient; sialagogue; stimulant; tonic; circulatory stimulant; expectorant; antiseptic; sexual tonic; anticatarrhal; antimicrobial; antiviral; hypoglycemic

Indications: Migraines; motion sickness; morning sickness; indigestion; flatulence; cough; cold; abdominal chills; bronchial/respiratory problems; cold extremities; poor peripheral circulation (hands and feet); menstrual cramps; rheumatism; fatigue; learning issues; mental fog

Contraindications: Do not us during pregnancy (because it is warming and moving). *Essential oil:* Dilute before using on skin; the powdered form can burn the esophagus. Do not use essential oil during pregnancy. Use in cold conditions, not when there is heat in the body.

Methods of Preparation and Dosage

Decoction: Use 1 to 5 fresh ginger slices per 1 cup (235 ml) water. Boil for 20 to 25 minutes.

Infusion: Use ½ to 1 teaspoon dried ginger per 1 cup (235 ml) water.

Tincture: Use 30 to 60 drops of tincture 3 times a day.

Poultice: Apply fresh, grated ginger on cramps and joints; cover with a clean cloth.

Essential Oil: Dilute in a carrier oil for massage.

PEPPERMINT

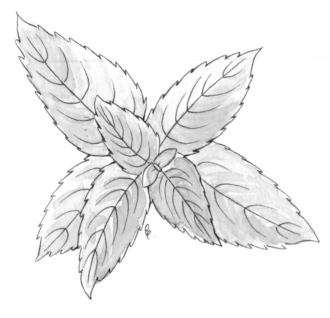

Every garden I have will always include peppermint! In African American spiritual traditions, we use peppermint to bring abundance you carry it in your wallet to ensure that you always have money. I use peppermint in my manifestation spells, placing it on my altar with my written desires to call in my greatest good. The plant is prolific and grows well under most circumstances. Its leaves are bright green and have multiple uses, all speaking to its spirit of abundance.

Peppermint is the most medicinal of all the mints. It stimulates our circulatory system while relaxing the nerves. It is brilliant at keeping the body calm and the mind stimulated, making us alert and clear. Peppermint moves you out of a mental fog, bringing you a clear head. I have used it as a head wash for confused thoughts, for assisting with the decision-making process, and as a compress for a headache. Rub peppermint essential oil diluted in a carrier oil onto the temples to manage irritability and stress.

Peppermint raises the vibration and clears any space. Use it as a floor wash to cleanse and remove unwanted energies or create a cleansing spray for you or your house. It can be burned as incense to enhance your psychic abilities and help you see a future where you achieve your desires. Peppermint is the best-tasting bitter I know! While its taste is not bitter, it functions in the digestive system as bitter.

Common Name: Peppermint

Latin Name: *Mentha* by *piperita*

Other Names: Mint

The Art & Practice of SPIRITUAL HERBALISM

Taxonomy: Lamiaceae

Botanical Description: Peppermint is a weedy, vigorous, creeping perennial, with purplish leaf margins and pink or purple flowers growing in a spike.

Native Habitat: Peppermint grows in temperate regions of the world. It is a hybrid created from a cross between spearmint and *Mentha arvensis.*

Wildcrafting and Cultivation: Grow by seed in the spring. It is best grown in a container, as it is a weed, and it will take over your garden! Harvest when not flowering. Peppermint likes full sun.

Parts Used: Leaves, flowering tops, essential oil

Planetary Influence/Correspondence: Mercury, Fire

Energetic Quality: Pungent, cool

Pharmacological Constituents: Volatile oils; menthol; flavonoids; rosmarinic acid; tannins; bitter principle; vitamins A and C; minerals; resin

Ethnobotanical/Historical Use: Peppermint was so valued in ancient Palestine that it was used to pay taxes. It has also had a history of use as a remedy for sexual dreams.

Actions/Properties: Amphoteric (stimulant to the circulatory system, relaxes nerves and organs); stimulant; dries dampness; carminative; cholagogue; antispasmodic; diaphoretic; antiemetic; nervine; analgesic; antimicrobial; antiseptic; alterative; expectorant

Indications: Mental fogginess; all digestion problems (except acid reflux); morning sickness; nausea; heartburn; fever; colds; insomnia; digestive headaches (when you wait too long to eat, or due to food allergies); stress; irritability; heart palpitations; irritable gallbladder; gallstones; coming off coffee; sore throat; toothaches

Contraindications: Do not use if you have acid reflux or with infants under two. Use spearmint instead. The essential oil can be used externally but must be diluted with a carrier oil.

Methods of Preparation and Dosage

Infusion: Use 1 tablespoon to 1 cup (235 ml) boiling water and drink up to 3 times a day.

Compress: Soak a cloth in a strong peppermint tea. Use a warm compress for pain and inflammation. Use a cold compress for itchy, burning conditions and for fever.

Bath and Steam: Peppermint leaves can be used in a bath, a foot soak, or a face steam for acne.

Hair/Head Rinse: Prepare a strong tea using 2 handfuls of mint leaves to 8 cups (1.9 L) water. Pour over your head in the shower. This stimulates the scalp and clears the head.

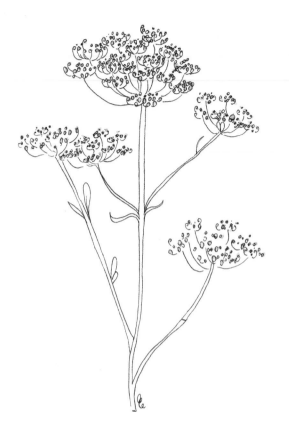

FENNEL

Fennel spiritual protection is strong and is used across Hoodoo and Voodoo practices to prevent and remove hexes. I often use fennel in a purification bath to clear negative energies and bring in protection. Fennel has a history of use to protect babies from "bad eye" or energy exchanges. For me that feels like fennel is protective of our most vulnerable selves from negative energetic exchanges.

I also use fennel to strengthen my physical and spiritual vision. It clears spiritual sight to see through the cloudiness of mental fog. I had a student compare fennel to Archangel Michael's energy, as its energy cuts through darkness to provide protection and clarity. Interestingly this plant has a history of being used for snow blindness (when the light of the Sun hits the snow and temporarily affects your vision).

Use fennel in a bath by infusing 7 tablespoons (40 g) in 7 cups (1.7 L) water for 20 to 25 minutes and adding it to your bathwater. Carry fennel with you in a mojo bag to enlist its protective energies. It also can be hung over your doorways or placed in corners to protect you and your home.

Common Name: Fennel

Latin Name: *Foeniculum vulgare*

Other Names: Sweet Fennel, Hinojo

Taxonomy: Apiaceae

Botanical Description: Fennel is a tall, clump-forming biannual with white to yellow flower heads that grow in umbels. The plant has a stem base that is a bulb. The leaves are alternating, feathery, and divided.

Native Habitat: Southern Europe; naturalized in America and Australia; cultivated in temperate regions worldwide

Wildcrafting and Cultivation: When wildcrafting, make sure you know your species. Gather seeds when the seed head turns brown. Sow seeds in rich, well-drained, sandy soil in late fall or January.

Parts Used: Seeds, whole plant, essential oil

Planetary Influence/Correspondence: Mercury, Fire

Energetic Quality: Pungent, acrid, sweet, warm, dry

Pharmacological Constituents: Volatile oil; coumarins; flavonoids; sterols; vitamins A and C; calcium; iron; zinc; magnesium; potassium; silicon; phosphorus; essential fatty acids

Ethnobotanical/Historical Use: Fennel was used in early medicine to bring surgical patients out of amnesia. Native people would use it as an antidote for witchcraft and snakebite. Historically it has also been used to stop hunger pangs.

Actions/Properties: Carminative; aromatic; digestive; anesthetic; tonic; appetite suppressant; anti-inflammatory; antibacterial; antispasmodic; galactagogue; hepatic; mild sedative for children; expectorant; emmenagogue; vermifuge; diuretic; improves vision; estrogenic

Indications: Fennel aids in the digestion of fatty foods and stabilizes blood sugar. Use for gas, indigestion, allergies, weak digestion, and bad breath. Helps with weight loss. Good for colic in babies. Brings in rich milk supply. Add to laxatives to ease stomach cramps. Assimilates nutrients. Decongestant for liver. Clears stagnation. Use for endometriosis, amenorrhea, low libido, hypertension, diabetes, and poor eyesight.

Contraindications: Do not use if you have acid reflux or estrogenic conditions in the body. During pregnancy, do not use strong fennel tea; instead, eat as food or add a few seeds to food.

Methods of Preparation and Dosage

Infusion: Crush the seeds with the back of the spoon before infusing. Use 1 tablespoon (6 g) per 1 cup (235 ml) boiling water. Let steep for 20 to 25 minutes.

Tincture: Use 30 to 60 drops of tincture 3 times a day.

Topically: Fennel can be used as an anti-inflammatory eyewash. Make the tea as stated above and use it to rinse the eye.

For Babies: To make gripe water, make a weak infusion. Use 1 teaspoon to 1 cup (235 ml) water and administer by the teaspoon every few hours.

ADDITIONAL PLANTS

Marshmallow *Althea officinalis*

Marshmallow dates to before Egyptian times, where this root was used as part of the mummification process, enabling the Spirit to travel safely to its destination. In Voodoo and Hoodoo medicine this herb is a spirit-puller to draw in good spirits. I have used marshmallow to heal a broken or stagnant connection between individuals and their ancestors.

Another important way I love to use marshmallow is to soften the will for those who honor their head over their heart—softening our approach to self and others. I find it tremendously helpful in developing compassion for self and self-forgiveness.

Marshmallow is the plant that lets us know that effective medicine does not have to be harsh. This velvety soft plant is a healer. It heals irritation and distress in any of our mucous membranes throughout our bodies. It heals irritated bronchial passages and is useful for many respiratory complaints, such as a harsh cough. It is also healing to the gastrointestinal tract and helpful for gastritis, ulcers, and acid reflux.

Contraindications: Do not use if you have profuse congestion. Marshmallow can slow the absorption of prescription medications.

Black Walnut *Juglans nigra*

A black walnut tree can live for over a thousand years. The energy of this tree is that of a wise grandfather. The medicine of the tree is strongly antiparasitic. Black walnut has been used to rid the body of parasitic infections, fungal infections, and candida. Under the influence of the Sun and Fire, this plant's energy is intense.

Legend says to receive a bag of walnuts is to see all your dreams come true and your wishes fulfilled. I use black walnut to weed out parasitic thoughts that stand between us and our wisdom and the vision we have for ourselves.

The Doctrine of Signatures shows us that the walnut, shaped like the brain, is indicated for all things related to the brain. Because of its high concentration of omega fatty acids, walnuts have shown that they protect the brain, increase cognitive function, and prevent age-related memory decline.

Contraindications: Black walnut is not for prolonged use. Juglone (one of its chemical components/constituents) has mutagenic properties. Do not use if pregnant or nursing.

Lemongrass *Cymbopogon citratus*

Lemongrass, or "fever grass," as we would call it in my home of Guyana, is an ancestral medicine. In the village of Essequibo, where I grew up, there was not a home garden that did not have fever grass. As a child, it was one of the first plants I knew how to identify positively. My grandmother would often send the children to gather plants we needed, and lemongrass was gathered before dinner to make into a hot tea to help with digestion. I still use it this way.

Lemongrass warms the digestive fire and warms up slow and sluggish digestion. Lemongrass is an excellent digestive nervine and antispasmodic, easing digestive discomfort and cramps and relaxing the gut's nerves to allow for proper food breakdown. Because of its warming properties, lemongrass is useful for fever and chills and removes mucus from the respiratory tract.

Contraindications: They are none. Lemongrass is considered safe for use.

Cardamom *Elettaria cardamomum*

Cardamom is another herb I use to demonstrate how we commonly use herbal medicines without recognizing that we are using herbs. Cardamom is a spice used to season foods worldwide, most notably in Southwest Asia and North African regions. How many of us have received cardamom after finishing a meal at a restaurant? I often point out how all our spices are medicinal, and we use herbal medicine each day to make our foods.

Cardamom, like fennel, is warm and dry and guided by Mercury. Mercurian plants are perfect for assisting with digestion. Many of them are spices. Cardamom aids in the breakdown of grains, increasing their digestibility, and is useful for celiac disease. It reduces stomach acidity and helps prevent gas, bloating, and cramps. Chewing on a few cardamom seeds improves your breath. This plant is useful to treat halitosis, which stems from poor digestion.

Contraindications: Cardamom is considered very safe. Use in food. Avoid cardamon with any gastrointestinal tract ulcers.

Bitthas! Digestive Bitters

Digestive bitters has a history of use across many cultures. They are used as a bitter tonic, an aperitif, or a tea before eating a meal. When I was growing up in Guyana, my mother often served a bitter cup of sweet broom tea with dinner. As a child, I remember that the taste changed everything following. I prefer to use a tonic/tincture instead of drinking a cup of tea because of the bitters' strength.

Bitters are essential to the digestive process. They prepare the stomach to receive food, and they signal the liver to release bile to break down our food. Many of the bitter herbs in this recipe are cholagogues, a substance that stimulates bile flow from the liver and gallbladder.

These bitters are best taken 20 minutes before eating on an empty stomach. You can prepare these bitters using double the amount of fresh herbs.

2 tablespoons (6 g) dried dandelion root

2 tablespoons (6 g) dried burdock root

2 tablespoons (4 g) dried peppermint leaves

1 tablespoon (6 g) dried yellow dock root

1 teaspoon dried gentian root

1 teaspoon dried orange peel

½ teaspoon cardamom pods

1 cup (235 ml) brandy

Yield: 8 ounces (227 g)

Place all the herbs in an 8-ounce (235 ml) wide-mouth mason jar. Cover entirely with the brandy. Label your medicine with the date, herbs, and brandy. Shake very well and place in a cool place out of direct sunlight. Shake your medicine each time you see it.

Let it sit for 4 to 6 weeks. After the herbs tincture, use a cheesecloth or fine-mesh strainer to strain off the plant material. Discard the used plant material. Store the tincture in a dark glass bottle with a dropper and label the bottle. Take 30 drops 20 minutes before eating on an empty stomach.

Store your medicine in a cool, dry space out of direct sunlight. Medicine made this way lasts about two years when stored correctly.

That Feeling Digestive Tea

Over the years of being an herbalist, I have learned there is always a reason to have a digestive tea handy. This formulary aids in after-dinner digestion. It supports food breakdown, and it alleviates indigestion, gas, and bloating. Sacred Vibes Apothecary has a similar blend that sells out each holiday when we all tend to eat large meals. I make a pot of this tea for my family on most nights after dinner.

2 tablespoons (4 g) dried chamomile flowers

1 tablespoon (4 g) dried peppermint leaves

1 teaspoon dried gingerroot

1 teaspoon fennel seeds, crushed

½ teaspoon cardamom pods

Honey (optional)

Yield: 5 cups (1.2 L)

Add all of the herbs to a large bowl. Pour 5 cups (1.2 L) boiling water over the herbs, cover, and let it infuse for 20 to 25 minutes. Strain off the plant material using a fine-mesh sieve and discard. Though I rarely need to sweeten this tea, some of my customers have added honey and loved it! Store any unused material in a glass jar out of direct sunlight.

Fresh and Clean Breath Spray

This breath spray is a simple and effective way to keep your breath fresh throughout the day! It is useful for keeping healthy bacteria in the mouth. There is much research that shows that our dental health and gut health are related. The bacteria in our mouth also live in our digestive tract. During the COVID-19 pandemic, we found that dental health informed our immune system responses to the virus.

I use essential oils when making this recipe; choose essential oils that are appropriate for internal use. This recipe uses no alcohol to preserve. Instead I rely on essential oils for preservation. The shelf life is a month, and I encourage you to remake it when needed.

2 ounces (60 ml) distilled water

5 drops peppermint essential oil

5 drops clove essential oil

Yield: 2 ounces (60 ml)

Pour the distilled water into a clean 2-ounce (60-ml) glass spray bottle. Add the drops of essential oil and shake well. Label the bottle and carry it with you. Spray directly in your mouth whenever needed. Store in a cool, dry place.

Laying Hands Stomach and Womb Oil

This is one of my favorite recipes. I have found it useful for minor constipation or indigestion after large meals. Use this oil over the womb area for menstrual discomfort and fibroid pain. I talk below about the ancestral art of laying of hands. This oil complements that practice. Use dry plant material to prepare the oil.

1 tablespoon (2 g) dried mugwort leaves

1 tablespoon (6 g) dried gingerroot

1 tablespoon (6 g) dried cinnamon pieces

1 tablespoon (5 g) dried cayenne powder

3 ounces (85 ml) olive oil

1 ounce (28 ml) castor oil

Yield: 4 ounces (120 ml)

Place all the plant material in a 4-ounce (120-ml) wide-mouth mason jar. Cover with the olive and castor oils. Label the jar with the date, herbs, and oils. Place in your sunniest window for 4 to 6 weeks. After that time, strain using a fine-mesh sieve. Discard the plant material and retain the oil. Store the oil in a clean and dry narrow-mouth glass jar and label. Please see the ritual practice opposite for recommended use.

Store oil in a dry place out of direct sunlight. This oil will last for 6 months.

Ritual Practice: Dismantling Beliefs: Laying of Hands

What beliefs around our worth and work have we internalized from our oppressors? As Black women, we especially hold beliefs throughout our lives that we were not the origin. We believe that we have to work hard, are not deserving, and have limited access to abundance. We grow up hearing, "Money doesn't grow on trees."

This ancestral ritual practice helps heal the damage of inherited familiar and institutionalized beliefs that reside in us. Through this practice, we dismantle and let go of our outgrown views that no longer serve our greatest good.

Black people have inherited spiritual technologies from our ancestors, which heal us. One such technology is the art of laying of hands. The hands direct powerful spiritual energy. Whether through mudras or Reiki symbols, the hands bring tremendous intention and healing to the body and spirit.

In African American culture, the practice of laying of hands has healed countless people from spiritual and physical illnesses. We know that the power of Grandma's hand is transformative. This power lies in your hands as well, waiting to awake. This practice will help. Do this with a partner or in your own company. This ritual uses the Laying Hands Stomach and Womb Oil (page 70).

The Laying of Hands

Begin by noticing for seven days the thoughts that come throughout the day, write them down, and try to recognize where they originate and whose belief system has governance. Is it your mother's, your partner's, your aunt's, your own? Write it down.

Each day choose a belief you want to let go of and do this practice of releasing.

Clean your hands, pour some oil into them, and vigorously rub your hands together while repeating, "These hands have the power to heal me!" Do this at least seven times until your hands have warmed.

Lay your hands gently on your belly, repeating your intention and asking for release.

Lean into your body and feel what it needs. Either move your hands in a circular clockwise motion or lay them still over whatever spot Spirit leads you. Feel the energy transfer from your warm hands to your body.

Visualize warm sunlight or the warmth of a steady fire pouring into your stomach through your hands, breaking through and eliminating any limiting beliefs.

Continue this practice for at least 7 minutes. When completed, wrap your belly and keep it warm for the remainder of the day. If possible, use an orange or yellow cloth; these are warm colors that support solar plexus healing.

Continue this practice for a full seven days and then burn the paper on which you wrote what you needed to release.

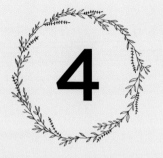

4

Nourishing Anger
LIVER HEALTH

———

In Chinese medicine the liver is the seat of anger in our bodies. All emotions find a home in our bodies, and the liver holds our rage. There are things happening around us that make us angry, and we will feel this necessary emotion. It is a misconception that spiritual people cannot or should not get mad. Many of us struggle to recognize and deal with anger on our spiritual path.

Anger is a catalyst to change. When nourished and directed, it motivates us to grow and create change for ourselves, our families, and our communities.

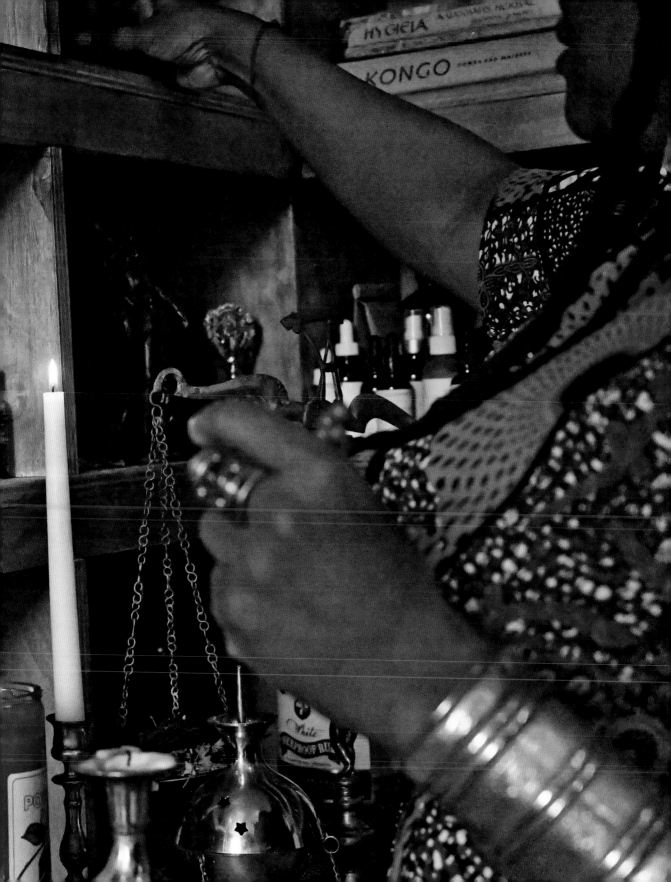

Like all our family legacies, anger is a legacy. How our family processes and deals with anger influences how we learn to process and deal with anger. The way that our family has dealt with anger is a legacy stored in our bodies. Sometimes we do the opposite of what our family has done, or sometimes we process our rage in the exact way we have seen and learned—carrying these dynamics into our lives. Once we know that we are replicating what our families have done, we try to manifest the opposite, some of us to no avail.

Denial of your family's legacy is not healthy, nor does it move you toward wholeness. You are your family, and you are those people. It is natural to repeat what they did. Healing takes acknowledgment of the legacy you have inherited. Often it takes work after you've moved to the opposite of your family's legacy to return to the middle. This work includes realizing that your anger is restorative and relearning how to process it.

Some families process social or political anger and decline to process interpersonal anger within the family. Some families process anger through addiction, emotional eating, and secrecy. Some families lash out or bottle it in, holding in anger and building resentment and then exploding in anger and holding the regret that follows. Many think if they don't verbally express or physically lash out, they are not angry. We pride ourselves on not being an angry person, someone who maintains themselves and remains silent.

What is more violent than silence? This behavior cuts others off. Your silence is violence to the self and others. When you are silent and angry, your actions are still that of anger. It breeds a lack of empathy and compassion, as well as fear, untruth, and inauthentic relationships. Silent rage finds its manifestation in the body. Inflammation, autoimmune issues, and thyroid conditions are an inflamed Spirit letting it out through the body.

To nourish and heal your relationship to anger, begin with your essential relationships. Extend empathy and sit with people and look at the whole of their situation. We could say that our parents are angry people. Looking deeper, we see that their anger is hereditary, and it comes from another generation. They are angry because their parents were angry, and their parents before them were angry and backward. Empathy means looking at the lineage of anger, traveling through generations, and noticing how it affects your family.

Empathy does not excuse the hurt caused. You may understand your history, but actions still hurt others. Your wound is valuable, and your anger is righteous and a catalyst for healing. Indigenous ancestral practice reminds us that when we heal ourselves, we are healing seven generations back and fourteen generations forward.

What I have noticed is when you do this healing work, your parents start to do the work, your siblings start to do the work, and it ripples throughout the family. They realize that you are not engaging

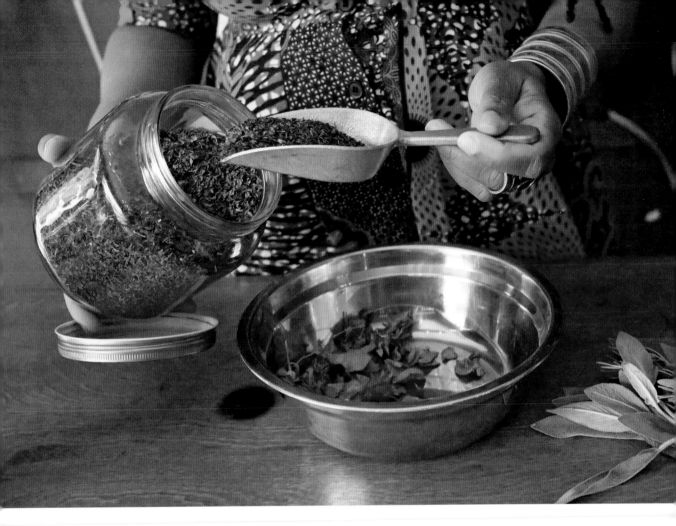

as you have done before, whether with silence, ignoring, or exploding. Their approach to you has to change if they choose to be in right relationship with you. As you change, other people around you will change.

Having a restorative practice of nourishing and honoring your anger includes learning what your needs are and how to be addressed and affirmed.

Understand the trauma you are still holding and how it influences your reactions. Learn how to move through these traumas by not judging yourself, but by giving yourself time and space, and by taking responsibility while building stronger, more authentic relationships.

The Spirit of the Liver

The liver, represented by Jupiter, the largest planet in our solar system, is a large, dynamic organ. Jupiter, known as the most benevolent planet, is about expansion, evolution, and the potential of our lives. Jupiter's energy asks you to view life as an adventure, an expression of yourself seeking growth and embracing the unknown. You were never meant to live a small life. Your life originated as a seed, and seeds grow and expand; they don't stay a seed. Your life's purpose is to grow. To grow requires courageous action, which comes through everyday practice. Meet yourself where you are. What are you ready for today? What is one decision you can make today from a place of courage? That's all it takes to start. Speak boldly about yourself and take up as much space as you need. Celebrate the people who do this well. Learn from their example and speak grandly of yourself.

Jupiter's energy parallels the energy of the orisha Obatala, the creator of life, and the orisha of the white cloth. Known for purity and universal truth, Obatala bestows health, justice, peace, and happiness. He imparts to us wisdom and discernment. The liver is responsible for the body's purity and, when functioning well, sends life-giving energy, our cleaned blood, to all our body's organs and structures, revitalizing our life. The liver is the only regenerative organ—it renews itself. It is the truth.

The first step to healing is always the truth. Being whole requires connecting to our vulnerability and telling ourselves the truth about our situation and ourselves. Take time to nourish, nurture, and love yourself through this process.

Getting in touch with the things that make us angry is a necessary step toward healing. Think of all the work we do to be nice. Our parents have raised nice people who are judged when angry. The nicest people are usually allergic to many things, and their skin breaks out regularly.

Our anger does not disappear. It shows up in our bodies. When we do not use our voice, the body speaks in other ways of our discomfort and anger. Our liver responds when there is a lack of emotional processing. The imbalance is on both sides, and this is true for both the person who explodes with anger regularly and the person who never expresses anger.

Telling the truth is consensual. Invite others into the reciprocal exchange of truthtelling. Give people space to live in their truth as you live in yours. If you are doing the work of calling in or out, be prepared to be a reflection. The moment you tell someone about their truth gives them space to tell you about yours. In this way we notice when we should be speaking and when we should not. Were you asked? Did you examine whether what's said may not be their truth, but rather the truth of how you perceive and receive that person?

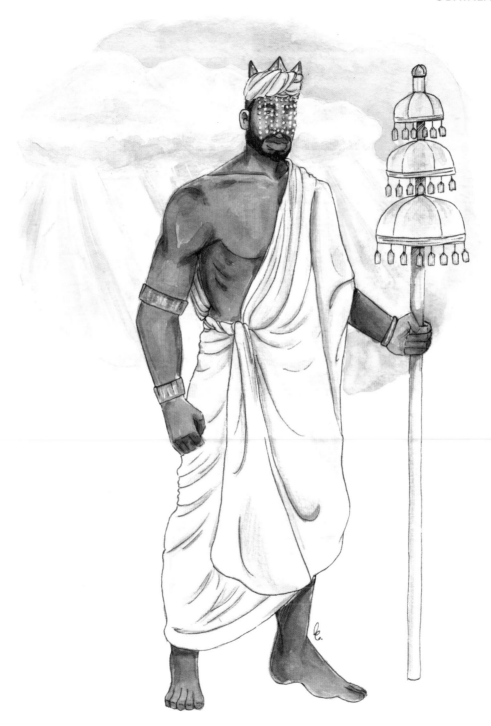

When you hear others' comments on your life and who they believe you are, process it, filter it, and eliminate it if it is not your truth. If it is not your truth, there is no need for you to hold on to it. When you do so, you grow a lack of ease. Live your truth, identify your life's purpose, and live it out. No one will give you the life you want. You are more than enough to create the life you desire.

Fear

Over the years I have asked my students: If your fear could talk, what would it say? Some answers have been: Don't mess up. You can't. You're not. That sounds hard. Keep yourself small. You are not capable, not good enough. You will fail. You didn't do that right. You didn't say that right. No one's going to like you. You will make people feel bad. Stay where you are. You are too broke, too ghetto, too Black, too fat. You're not normal. I don't know. I can't. My ideas are too big, too much. It's too late. I should feel guilty. How dare I. Be quiet. I don't deserve to be here. I haven't done enough. They are all right; what have *you* done?

It is essential to know how your fear speaks, so you can hear it when it's talking to you. Fear has a specific voice, and you have to realize that voice. When you don't know what fear sounds like and how it speaks to you, all your decisions come from that place. Your life is then a life based on fear. Think about how many decisions you have made in the last few months that were fearbased. In your daily decisions about your life, do you consciously or unconsciously confirm that voice? As a mother of two Black boys going out into the world each day, I have to recognize fear's voice in my head to make decisions from a place of love and life. My boys deserve to live their life expansively.

For some of us, fear is our consistent voice. Notice the decisions you make because you have chosen to live small. When you find yourself worried about the outcome before taking action, identify where fear might be holding you back from living your truth. Say to your fears, "I see you, I know who you are, I can hear you, and I acknowledge when you show up. I can feel how my body responds to you." The voice of fear shows up in your body's responses. Notice how your muscles tighten, your stomach flutters, your heart races.

Many of us operate under someone else's fear. People will ask us, "Are you sure?" After listening to them, we aren't sure anymore. Our parents may have been afraid to do things. Their ancestors were afraid to do more things, and their ancestors before that were even afraid to read and write. We come from that legacy, where our fears can now originate. When making plans to accomplish your life's purpose, it's crucial to pay attention to who you let in: Sometimes we share our dreams with folks who are fearful and cannot imagine or support our dreams because of their fears. These are not the people to tell about your plans. We need folks to talk to who use discernment and move us ahead to the next best step.

The gallbladder works in tandem with the liver and houses fear. These two organs are in a relationship with each other, as are anger and fear. The gallbladder stores what the liver gives it, and likewise, fear builds deep-seated anger. The saying "You have so much gall!" comes directly from the function of the gallbladder. How dare you have the audacity? Or the gall? To have gall means that you will live an expansive, whole life.

Any organ not fully utilized atrophies. The number of women having their gallbladder removed is significantly higher than other genders. Think about the history of women and gall. How many of us could live in our audacity? How many Black women live with gall? We live in a culture that doesn't encourage women to be audacious and daring. Decide to tap into the courage of your ancestors and demonstrate your gall. Support yourself by pushing your limits, pushing boundaries, and having the gall to do the things that are important to you; whether or not the outcome is uncertain or unknown, take a risk.

Gratitude

Gratitude is a quick way to nourish and heal anger and resentment. Be grateful for your life, for the things in your world that are working for you. Be thankful for the wounded people who brought you here. Find whatever it is that you are grateful for, attach gratitude to it, and repeat it to yourself as a practice.

The moment you express gratitude, more comes into your life. The best attraction magnet is gratitude. The more grateful you are, the more goodness you attract. Be thankful for your body and your breath. Have a daily gratitude practice. Write one thing you are grateful for each night. This may sound so simple, yet it works so well. This practice reminds us as we go to sleep to be in a place of thanksgiving; that one thing we are thankful for carries us through the night and into the next morning.

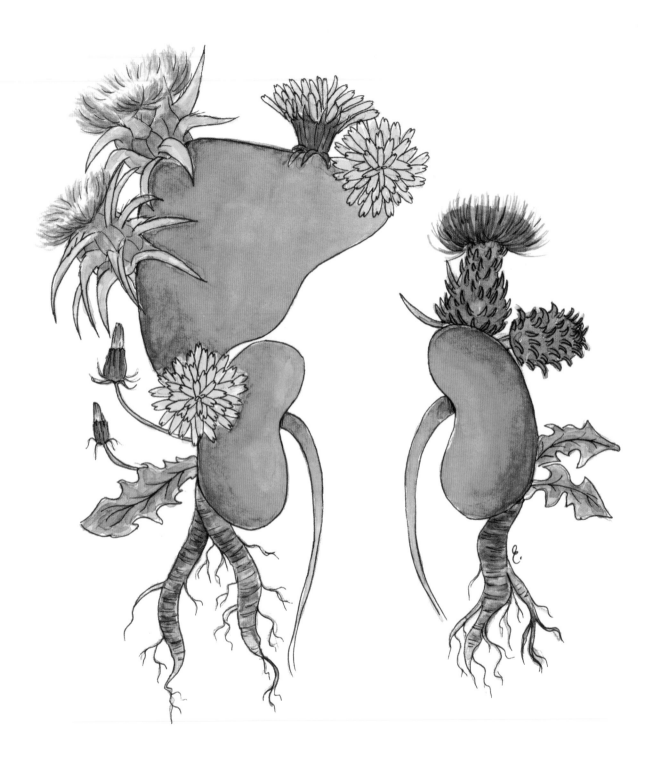

The Art & Practice of SPIRITUAL HERBALISM

The Liver

Though part of the digestive system, the liver is so essential to the body's function that I have decided to cover it independently. Along with the gallbladder, the liver plays a vital role in the detoxification of the body. Our liver has to process everything that we take in, including environmental toxins, the air we breathe, the water we drink, and the metabolic wastes coming from our body's cells. Pharmaceutical and over-the-counter drugs also have to be processed by the liver.

In constant diligence, our liver filters more than 2 quarts (2 L) of blood each minute. Hormonal balance, beautiful skin, a healthy digestive system, and reproductive health require healthy liver function. All our organs are fed a clean, oxygen-rich blood supply from the liver. When excess toxins overburden the liver, the primary organ of elimination, then the body's other elimination organs—our colon, kidneys, lungs, and skin—have to work harder to compensate.

Our bodies are our best teachers, and what occurs physically parallels what is occurring spiritually. The liver's work is to process, store, filter, and eliminate spiritually. As the liver processes toxins from the body, it also processes our emotions. As it filters, it requires us to filter our experiences and know the truth, hold and store wisdom, and eliminate—let go of that which no longer serves us. Unprocessed anger can lead to developing habits and addictions. Long-seated anger shows symptoms of heat in the body and come out as issues with our skin: eczema and psoriasis, systemic inflammation, and immune dysfunction. Anger also presents as a backup of toxins in the digestive system, triggering gut issues and bad breath.

Plants for the Liver

Over the years I have given my customers our detox liver tea, and they have returned to the shop wanting to know why they spent the last few days mad at everyone. They return, demanding to know what we gave them. I usually ask them to buy some more tea because obviously, this process is not over. When using plants that support the liver, your liver releases, and yes, anger surfaces; when this happens, you will speak on things you have been carrying for some time.

BURDOCK

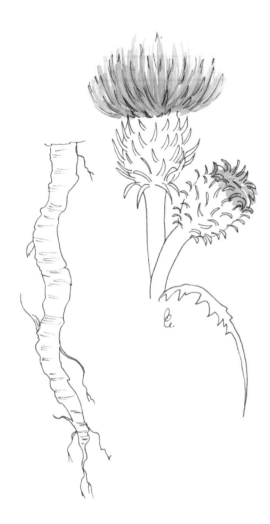

Burdock is a plant of Venus and holds the mirror of truth, helping us see the beauty of the truth. It reveals the truth about us and our deep-rooted subconscious beliefs, habits, and emotions. In my practice, we call burdock "truth serum." Over the years, my apprentices have recognized that a walk with burdock is never an easy one.

Burdock is a taproot plant, growing deep into the soil, touching the ancestors' realm. It is ready to dig into buried trauma and the truth of old wounds. Its magic is to bring this wounding to the surface, that we may heal. Often when we first take burdock, we encounter a "healing crisis," where the condition worsens over the first few days and then becomes better. It is this way that burdock also works spiritually. The wound has to reveal itself to heal.

Burdock is especially good at breaking up and releasing old habits. It helps us examine the truth behind the pattern, which can be uncomfortable. Through the healing process, this medicine grounds us deeply, unveiling fears and unresolved emotions, rooting us in the truth.

Common Name: Burdock

Latin Name: *Arctium lappa*

Other Names: Bardana, Beggar's Button, Burr Seed

Taxonomy: Asteraceae

Botanical Description: Burdock is a robust perennial plant, with coarse stems, large leaves with a wool-like underside, and purple thistle flowers. Burdock has a taproot that grows as deep as 6 feet (1.8 m) into the soil.

Native Habitat: Europe; parts of Asia and North America

Wildcrafting and Cultivation: Sow seeds in fall or late winter. Gather during the first year, in spring, after it rains.

Parts Used: Roots, seeds, leaves

Planetary Influence/Correspondence: Venus, Water

Energetic Quality: Bitter, sweet

Pharmacological Constituents: Amino acids; inulin; carbohydrates; minerals; essential oils

Ethnobotanical/Historical Use: Burdock was pounded into wine to treat leprosy in the fourteenth century.

Actions/Properties: Alterative; diaphoretic; diuretic; antitumor; antiphlogistic; bitter; stool softener; antibacterial; antiarthritic; demulcent; vulnerary; nutritive; tonic; slow, but deep and sure

Indications: Skin eruptions; acne; eczema; psoriasis; gout; heart conditions; boils; inflammation; cancer; edema; chemical exposure; PMS; kidney problems; toxic buildup; alcohol, drug, and smoking use; blood cleanser; spring cleansing herb

Contraindications: Burdock lowers blood pressure. For people taking insulin with diabetes, it can lower blood sugar levels.

Methods of Preparation and Dosage

Decoction: Simmer 1 teaspoon in 2 cups (475 ml) water for 20 to 25 minutes. Begin with 1 cup (235 ml) per day for the first 2 weeks, then increase to 2 cups (470 ml) daily. Burdock is a tonic plant used over 3 months at a time as needed.

Tincture: Use 30 to 60 drops of tincture 3 times a day.

As Food: Purchase gobo/burdock root at your greengrocery and add it to broths and soups.

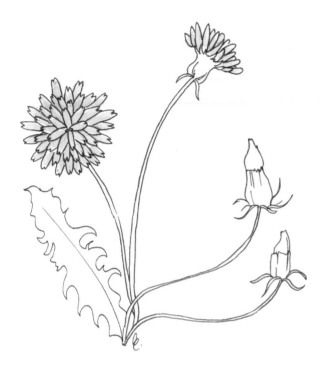

DANDELION

Dandelion's common name is lion's tooth. I use this to draw an analogy: When fed, a lion is satiated and calm. When hungry, that calm disappears. When we are angry, we are much like a hungry lion. When we are not being fed, heard, seen, and appreciated, our anger feels like a roar, with truths that can devour.

Dandelion is the expression of truth. The leaves have jagged edges, much like how truth feels jagged—truths are rarely smooth. The truth is a baseline when learning how to heal from unexpressed anger and its manifestations in the body.

The plant grows directly from the root—truth from the issue's source, with directness. This herb helps build the relationship to your voice, where you show up for yourself and say what you need to say. Dandelion builds confidence and the courage to express grief, dispersing your true feelings. Use dandelion to speak your truth even when you might not have it smoothly outlined in your mind.

The myth of using the blowball of a dandelion flower dispersed by your breath to get your wishes met is associated with the Air element. Dandelion, guided by Mercury, governs the voice. Having a strong voice and confidently speaking your desires into the Universe is how you get your wishes met.

Common Name: Dandelion

Latin Name: *Taraxacum officinale*

Other Names: Blowball, Lion's Tooth, Pissin Lit, Wild Endive

Taxonomy: Asteraceae

The Art & Practice of SPIRITUAL HERBALISM

Botanical Description: Dandelion is a perennial with a thick taproot. The root has latex in it and springs from a basal rosette of leaves, with bright yellow flowers that grow directly from the ground. Its puffball seed heads turn into blowballs.

Native Habitat: Greece; Arabia; Asia Minor; naturalized across the world in northern temperate regions

Wildcrafting and Cultivation: Dandelion is rarely cultivated for medicinal uses because it springs up everywhere. Find a patch in clean soil to harvest. The plant can be grown from seed, and it grows like a weed.

Parts Used: Root, leaf, flower

Planetary Influence / Correspondence: Jupiter, Air

Energetic Quality: Bitter, sweet, cool

Pharmacological Constituents: Tannins; inulin; polysaccharides; 7,000 units of vitamin A per ounce (28 g); calcium; magnesium; iron; leaves are rich in potassium

Ethnobotanical/Historical Use: Roasted dandelion root is used as a coffee substitute. In the seventh century, dandelion wine was used to treat liver and digestion issues.

Actions/Properties: Diuretic; hepatic; cholagogue (releases bile); laxative; tonic; bitter; nutritive; alterative; choleretic (produces bile); galactagogue; hypotensive; cleanses, nourishes, and supports the liver. *Leaf:* Water retention (edema) in any part of the body. *Root:* Liver congestion; inflammation; autointoxication.

Indications: *Root:* Jaundice; liver congestion; cirrhosis of the liver; hepatitis; adult-onset diabetes; blood disorders; eczema; psoriasis; rheumatism; gout. *Leaf:* Anemia; nutritional deficiencies; water retention in edema; PMS.

Contraindications: Do not use in cases of intestinal obstruction, blockage of the bile duct, bile duct cancer, or acute stomach inflammation.

Methods of Preparation and Dosage

Decoction: Simmer 1 teaspoon of root in 2 cups (475 ml) water for 20 to 25 minutes. Drink ½ cup (120 ml) 2 times a day. Build up to 1 cup (235 ml) after 2 weeks.

Infusion: Steep 1 tablespoon (3 g) dried leaves in 1 cup (235 ml) water for 25 minutes. Drink ½ cup (120 ml) 2 times a day. After 2 weeks, build up to 1 cup (235 ml), 2 times a day.

Tincture: Use 30 to 60 drops of tincture 2 times a day.

As Food: Use leaves in salad or fresh juice.

External Applications: The latex in the root can be used for beestings, sores, blisters, and warts.

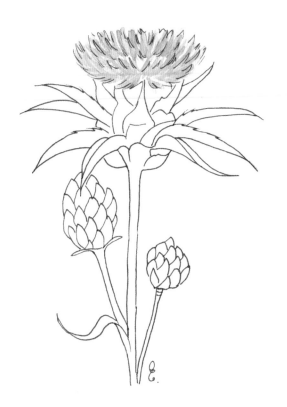

MILK THISTLE

Milk thistle, guided by the tremendous protective energy of Mars, protects us when we are most vulnerable, serving as protection from toxic situations and people. It establishes protection for those who have a habit that does not support their lives—such as overuse of food, substances, relationships, or sex.

Milk thistle teaches dedication, discipline, and appreciation, all qualities we need when healing a legacy of generational anger. It has a relationship to the Virgin Mary and offers compassion, holding you through self-forgiveness and repentance work. It offers renewal and regeneration, and protection while breaking curses.

Common Name: Milk Thistle

Latin Name: *Silybum marianum*

Other Names: Marian's Thistle, Our Lady's Thistle

Taxonomy: Asteraceae

Botanical Description: Milk thistle is a cultivated annual with a basal rosette of green leaves that are white marbled and deeply lobed with spiny margins. It has a purple thistle-like flower.

Native Habitat: Southwest Europe; Russia; North Africa; cultivated everywhere

Wildcrafting and Cultivation: Gather seeds when flowering puffs open and let dry. Plant in moist soil, 6 inches (15 cm) apart, in partial sun.

Parts Used: Seeds

Planetary Influence/Correspondence: Mars, Fire

Energetic Quality: Bitter, sweet, cool

Pharmacological Constituents: Bioflavonoids; silybin; bitter principle; polysaccharides; flavonoids

Ethnobotanical/Historical Use: Myth has it that the white lines on the leaves are from the tears of the Virgin Mary. It is an old remedy for melancholy. The unopened flower heads can be cooked like artichokes.

Actions/Properties: Hepatic protector; galactagogue; antioxidant; tonic; nutritive; alterative; stimulant; increases T-cell production; antiviral; antidepressant. Best liver protector there is!

Indications: Congestion in the liver, spleen, kidneys, and pelvic region; chronic skin problems; chronic allergies; jaundice; cirrhosis of the liver; hepatitis; alcoholism; acetaminophen poisoning; mushroom poisoning; exposure to internal and external toxins; protects and repairs damaged liver

Contraindications: None

Methods of Preparation and Dosage

Ground Seeds: Sprinkle the ground seeds on food or take 1 teaspoon per day in divided doses (⅓ teaspoon per dose). Ground seeds last for 10 days in the fridge.

Tincture: Use 30 to 60 drops of tincture 3 times a day.

Capsules (of ground seeds): Take 3 times a day.

ADDITIONAL PLANTS

Yellow Dock Root *Rumex crispus*

Here is a plant that the Doctrine of Signatures demonstrates well. The yellow in yellow dock root matches the bile produced in our livers, cleansing our bodies. Yellow dock root is a choleretic, aiding the release of bile from the liver.

Yellow dock is guided by Jupiter—the planet associated with potential and expansion. It mirrors this generosity by blessing us with abundance. Historically, spiritual uses included fertility and money spells. One of my spiritual teachers instructed me to mop my apothecary with yellow dock decoction to ensure abundant customers and sales. In Hoodoo traditions yellow dock root powder sprinkled in the far left-hand side of your home or house lot, known as the money corner, will ensure abundance.

Yellow dock is one of my favorite plants to treat eruptive skin issues such as eczema and psoriasis stemming from an overburdened liver. This plant treats a sluggish or fatty liver, slow digestion or constipation, and hemorrhoids. It is one of the best supports for anemia, building and increasing iron uptake in the blood without causing constipation. Use it to increase a low blood count during pregnancy.

Contraindications: Yellow dock should not be used breastfeeding mothers; do not use in cases of gout, kidney stones, or gallstones.

Sarsaparilla *Smilax officinalis*

Sarsaparilla is native to tropical America and the West Indies. There is no way you can travel to the Caribbean and not hear about this plant when asking about plant medicines. It is legendary and many traditional stories begin with sexual virility and having a "strong back" to perform sexual feats. Though sarsaparilla is excellent for sexual health, it is indicated for liver and kidney health, which feeds our sexual health.

Containing steroidal saponins, a hormonal precursor, sarsaparilla balances the hormones, especially in male bodies, explaining its use as an aphrodisiac. It is a potent blood cleanser and anti-inflammatory. It breaks down and releases any toxic buildup and addresses skin issues and joint inflammation.

Contraindications: Do not use during pregnancy or steroid therapy. Do not use in cases of kidney disease or gastric ulcers.

The Art & Practice of SPIRITUAL HERBALISM

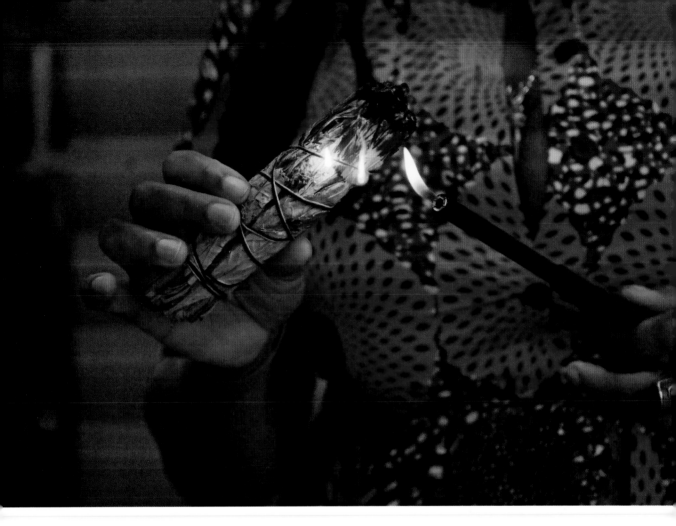

Schisandra Berries
Schisandra chinensis

Schisandra berries are ancestral medicine. They have a history of use in China for thousands of years. Commonly called the five taste berry, schisandra restores balance to our body's chi, or energy force, and is lifegiving and renewing.

Schisandra is a liver tonic and liver restorative, similar to milk thistle. It is an adaptogen and is used to treat liver disorders, such as hepatitis C, hormonal imbalances, and low immune function.

Contraindications: Do not use during pregnancy, in cases of epilepsy, or in conditions of too much heat, such as inflammation and rashes.

Heart Truth Burdock Hawthorn Vinegar

One of my favorite ways to administer nutritive-dense tonic herbs is through vinegar preparation, where vinegar is the menstruum rather than alcohol. Historically we have used tablespoons of vinegar to alkalize the blood, cleanse and tone the kidneys, release toxins from the body, and remove mucus and inflammation. Vinegar is versatile and can be used as a salad dressing or in cooking. I love the taste so much I have to remind myself to dose medicinally!

Burdock vinegar is something we make in early spring and take throughout the year as a cleansing tonic. I have included hawthorn in this recipe because if you have been taking burdock over a long period, you will see the need for heart-centeredness, which hawthorn so beautifully provides (see page 46). Burdock's lifting of the veil to our most profound truths can be an emotional ride. Leaning into hawthorn for heart and nervous system support creates synergy and encourages healing at the deepest level.

You can make this recipe with fresh or dried burdock root and hawthorn berries. When using freshly harvested plants, double the quantities of plants in the recipe.

3 tablespoons (9 g) dried burdock root	1 cup (235 ml) organic apple cider vinegar
3 tablespoons (26 g) dried hawthorn berries	**Yield:** 1 cup (235 ml)
1 tablespoon (3 g) dried gingerroot	

Place your herbs in a clean, sanitized 8-ounce (235 ml) wide-mouth mason jar with a plastic lid. It is essential to find a jar with a plastic lid; vinegar corrodes metal, and you will not be able to open your jar after it sits. Pour the apple cider vinegar over your plants and give it several good shakes. Place your medicine in a cool, dark place for 4 to 6 weeks. Shake your medicine each time you see it.

When it's ready, strain off the plants using a fine-mesh strainer. Discard the plant material. Decant the strained vinegar into a clean glass bottle, label, and store. Take this medicine by diluting 1 tablespoon (15 ml) in water and drinking 2 to 3 times a day.

Store in a cool, dark place out of direct sunlight. Vinegar extracts have an approximate 1-year shelf life.

Liver Support Tea

Many of our traditional foods are bitter and encourage cleansing. If you introduce bitters to your diet by drinking bitter teas, you will find that your taste for bitters will improve significantly after a month. The bitter taste of liver support tea is necessary for bile to be released into the blood to remove toxins.

The herbs in this formula—burdock, dandelion, and sarsaparilla—support liver function, and they are cholagogues and choleretics that build and encourage bile flow. This tea assists the body's detoxification process. Please note: When we release old toxins, we release old emotions, and tears will flow. Support yourself if necessary by taking other plant medicines to ease the heart (see page 8).

1 tablespoon (3 g) burdock root	1 tablespoon (9 g) schisandra berries
1 tablespoon (3 g) dandelion root	½ tablespoon gingerroot
1 tablespoon (3 g) sarsaparilla root	**Yield:** 3½ cups (825 ml)

Combine the herbs in a pot and cover them with 4 cups (940 ml) water. Bring to a boil and simmer for 25 minutes over low heat. Using a fine-mesh strainer, strain off the plant material and discard. You should end up with about 3½ cups (825 ml) of tea. Store the tea in a clean glass jar in the refrigerator.

Begin by drinking ¼ cup (60 ml), 2 times a day, on the first day. Increase that dosage to ½ cup (120 ml), 2 times a day, for the next 2 days. Finally move to 1 cup (235 ml), 2 times a day, to finish the jar.

A Castor Oil Pack for Liver Health

Using castor oil packs is a time-tested remedy for breaking up and removing stagnation in our joints and organs. Castor oil is applied topically to remove pain and swelling due to sprains and bruises. This recipe recommends castor oil to assist with the kidney and liver detoxification process. Castor oil increases the flow of lymph throughout the body and supports detoxification at the cellular level, improving organ function.

I infuse the castor oil with cinnamon and ginger to increase warmth and improve the detoxification process. I use this recipe as part of my spring detox routine. It is helpful whenever you are working on a kidney or liver detox and would like additional support.

4 cinnamon sticks	2 cups (475 ml) castor oil
½ cup (12 g) dried gingerroot	**Yield:** 2 cups (475 ml)

Pound your cinnamon sticks into small pieces using a mortar and pestle. Add the cinnamon and gingerroot to a clean 16-ounce (475 ml) mason jar and cover with the oil. Shake several times and place in a sunny window for 4 weeks. Shake the jar regularly.

After 4 weeks, using a clean cheesecloth, strain off the plant material from the oil. Discard the plant material. Store the oil in a clean glass bottle and label.

How to Use a Castor Oil Pack: Use a clean piece of cotton or wool cloth big enough to cover your body's desired area. Cutting up and reusing an old T-shirt works well.

Place about 1 cup (235 ml) of infused castor oil in a bowl (with a lid). Soak the cloth in the oil, making sure it's well saturated.

Apply the cloth to the skin right over the area of your body that you're addressing. Cover with a plastic sheet to keep the oil from staining your clothes.

Place a towel and a heating pack over the area and relax for at least 1½ hours.

When done, remove the cloth and store the cloth in the closed container in the refrigerator. When you are ready for the next use, let the cloth come to room temperature before.

Continue this practice for the next 3 to 5 days during your liver detox.

Ancestral Practice: Getting to Liberation

One year when relaxing at home in my native Guyana, this practice occurred to me. I found it enlightening and healing. I couldn't believe how effective it was at seeing the truth about my life. Seeing the truth is never easy, and as stated before, it is the best place to begin healing.

When doing this practice, be sure to take your time and write for as long as you need. Review this practice often. It keeps us connected to the root of our fears, the lies we have been living under, and the truth that will set us free. Notice where these fears are ancestral and place an offering on your ancestral altar along with a prayer to release them. One prayer I have found most helpful throughout the years is "I am free" and "I am free from fear." Let this be your mantra several times a day to remind you that you deserve to be free and liberated.

Meditative Writing Practice

This practice can be combined with the castor oil pack (see page 92).

Find a comfortable place to be alone and vulnerable with your thoughts in a peaceful environment. Use a favorite notebook and pen. I have found it helpful to connect to beauty when doing this exercise.

On a sheet of paper, draw three columns, and title them Fear, Lie, and Truth.

In the Fear column, list the fears you are carrying. They can be things such as "I will be alone" or "I will be poor."

In the next column, under Lie, examine and write the lie behind this fear.

For example, Fear: "I will be alone." Lie: "I will be alone without the love I deserve, or I can survive alone."

Fear: "I will be poor." Lie: "I deserve to be poor" or "I made the choices, and I am paying for them."

Now get to the truth. Under the Truth column, write the truth about reality as it exists. "I will be alone." now translates to "I am never alone. I cannot survive and thrive alone, and I have support systems around me and the support of Spirit and my ancestors."

"I am poor" now gets you the truth that everyone deserves abundance. "My choices don't define my life, and I make new choices each day."

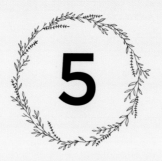

5

Standing in Your Power
SEXUAL HEALTH

———

Having a general understanding of fundamental sexual health concerns and knowing how to treat them is empowering. An impetus for my healing journey was understanding my body and knowing that I could heal myself, not turn my power over to a doctor to tell me what was happening in my body. It's essential to know our own anatomy.

Women and, more so, Black women have not been able to put their trust in the Western medical-industrial complex. There is a deep distrust of medical practitioners, knowing that we were experimented on to "advance" medicine. Lack of cultural competency among practitioners, poor cross-cultural communication, and language that disenfranchises patients seeking care create further barriers. Existing models of care ignore the unique legacy of Black bodies. There is no consideration of the effects of generational/ancestral/historical trauma held in Black bodies and spirits. Likewise there is no acknowledgment that Black women are more than their trauma and gifted with resilience in our physical and emotional bodies that translates into our existence.

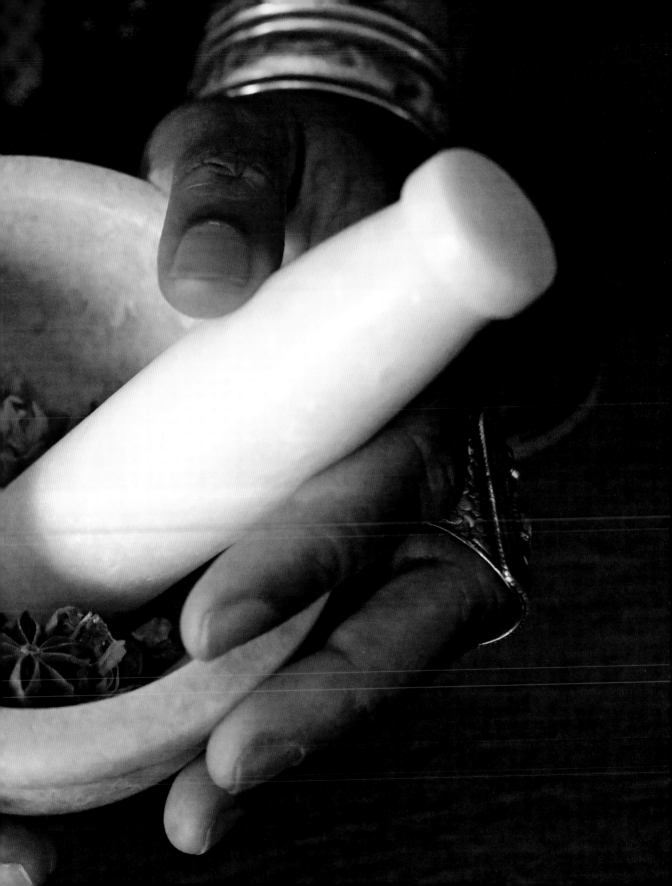

Complicating the invisibility of women's bodies, we live in a world where our reproductive and sexual health is seen through the lens of patriarchy or not spoken of at all. Black women and femmes particularly are oversexualized or ignored.

Despite Western medicine's many advancements, gynecological treatment has not grown at the same speed. Studies in this area are not heavily funded. As an indigenous herbalist, I am grateful to the midwives and wisewomen who have come before me who have assisted women through all life stages and have provided me a rich source of information on healing women's bodies.

Traditional education models have played a role in our disconnection from our sexual selves and sexual health. We may have had sexual education in high school, yet most of us left high school without a proper understanding of our sexual health.

It is essential with any sexual health issue that we are the ones who can initially identify that something isn't right, and we can seek care promptly. Empower yourself by understanding your body and its symptoms. It was crucial to me when I had my daughter Lauren to teach her to identify her body parts. When she said something was not feeling right, she would say that it was her ovary, her womb, or her cervix.

Stand in your power. Be the authority over your body. Healing is becoming comfortable with describing to caregivers what's happening in your body. Know when there is a lack of balance in your sexual health system, such as when you have a yeast or bacterial infection. Know what your discharge looks like, smells like, and tastes like, and the changes that occur throughout the month. We can become aware of these symptoms before going to the doctor and then walk into our doctor's offices empowered with information ready to share.

Trauma, Sexual Health, and Pleasure

I acknowledge that speaking about our sexual health can be triggering. This work is to open the door and create a space for you to inhabit when ready. I also acknowledge that my use of the word *trauma* might not be how you associate the experiences your body holds. Please feel free to name those experiences as you like.

The reproductive and sexual health system is part of the entire body, part of our Spirit, and part of our whole. Our whole self should be striving to have health. Various forms of sexual, emotional, and physical trauma can leave us feeling disconnected from our bodies. Surgery to our sexual organs or reproductive system might leave us recovering and healing from a traumatic experience. I have conversations with people who have said that the top half of their body feels disconnected from the bottom half of their body, functioning as two halves. They say that it's tough to get in touch with the bottom half. This feeling is especially true if they have experienced trauma. Many disassociate from their bodies to survive. I often meet these individuals when they decide to hold life and have a baby. They realize that it is challenging for new life to begin without a connection to our entire body.

I often speak publicly about vaginal health and witness the reactions around the room. Talking about the vagina or sexual health can bring anxiety and panic or resurface a memory of a traumatic experience. A few years back, I wrote a blog post on vaginal steaming. I received so much negative feedback from many whose relationships to their bodies and pleasure were shaped by the notion that the vagina is pristine and should never be touched, least of all by us. Vaginal steaming has been a practice since before Christianity, yet cultural and religious practices influence the way we view our bodies, specifically our sexual organs.

The practice of pleasure often involves reclaiming autonomy over the self and body—a reintroduction to yourself and your sexual power. Feeling safe and comfortable within your body is the first step. The practice of being embodied is often aided by self-pleasure and touch, as you are the most informed person to define what pleasure means to you. Leaning into pleasure and building a relationship with your body gives you the tools to translate that to another person. It is a conscious choice to prioritize pleasure.

Ancestral Connection

At birth, if you are born with ovaries, you hold all the eggs you will have in your lifetime, which means that we have already seeded our grandchildren. When my daughter was born, she had all the eggs she will ever carry, and therefore, I was holding her and her children in my womb. Both Lauren and her children would inherit whatever I was experiencing.

When I started teaching about sexual health more than twenty-three years ago, and I would speak of ancestral trauma, spiritual folks understood; scientific minds did not. Indigenous people have recognized that if our grandmothers experienced trauma, so did we. The egg that would become you was already a part of her at that time. Intergenerational trauma is the passing of this memory and fear, the same way we pass on our hair and eyes. Why wouldn't this translate? If they can track our brilliance to our DNA, why not also our trauma?

As a self-identified woman, I understood this right away on such a deep level as my practice grew. Many women expressed that they felt trauma, even though they had no memory of personal trauma in their life. It felt like an old wound coming back to haunt them. Healing, then, does not only encompass your life. It's about healing trauma backward and forward. Our healing informs generations of enslaved and oppressed people.

Womb health and healing are multifaceted. Your womb is a direct channel to your birthright, your innate or ancestral wisdom. Emotional baggage from relationships that existed years ago, or the trauma we come into this life with, or that we have acquired, block or close these channels. A healed womb is a portal to cosmic travel, where we can reach back to our ancestors' suffering and heal, and likewise, we can go forward to our children and heal them.

The Spirit of Sexual Health

Our sexual health, guided by the Moon and Pluto, is the orishas Yemaya and Shango's energy. Having strong planets in our birth chart ruled by the Moon or Pluto requires special attention to our sexual health. Many people with Scorpio as their Sun, Moon, or rising sign have identified sexual health issues.

Our sexual organs live at our base, or root, chakra, which is about survival and trust. Here at our root is where the powerful energy of Shango lives. Shango's energy is the nature of sexual power, kundalini energy. It is the most fertile energy we can use to tap into and birth our desires. Learning to dance with Shango's drumbeat or mastering our sexual energy liberates us from trauma and enhances our sexuality and pleasure.

Whenever trauma impacts our base or root, we feel unsafe and insecure. Feeling insecure, we move to control what will happen next. Our body desires to be vulnerable and liberated, and when we seek to control everything in our lives, imbalances like fibroids, delayed menses, and cysts may manifest. The base/root chakra corresponds to our throat chakra and asks us how vulnerable we are with our words, speaking the truth, communicating from the heart, and asking for our desires.

The power of the dark feminine, represented by Kali, also represents Pluto and is the power and mystery rooted in transforming the egoic self. Kali calls us to notice when the ego's energy shows up outwardly, often as fear, doubt, and manipulation. Are we involved in relationships where we don't feel powerful? Are we sharing power and having power with our partners instead of over our partners? Manipulation in partnerships takes from our sexual energy and creates an imbalance in power and our hormones. This imbalance of power can also show up in our work relationships. Many women of color end up in violent work relationships where microaggressions and patriarchy dominate. When our work pressures begin to demonstrate in our bodies, it is often within the sexual health and reproductive system.

Learning to balance power and living with a spirit of release and forgiveness are critical issues in our sexual health. Paradoxically, zodiac signs with the energy of Water—Cancer, Pisces, and Scorpio—may find releasing challenging. They might struggle to allow the authentic self to lead and let go of things or people that no longer serve them. Questions to ask ourselves are: Who would I be if I were free? What does liberation mean for me and those with whom I am in relationship?

The Art & Practice of SPIRITUAL HERBALISM

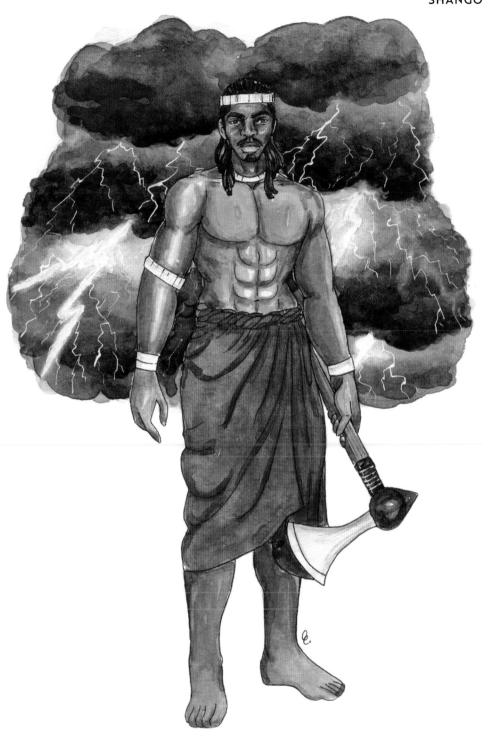

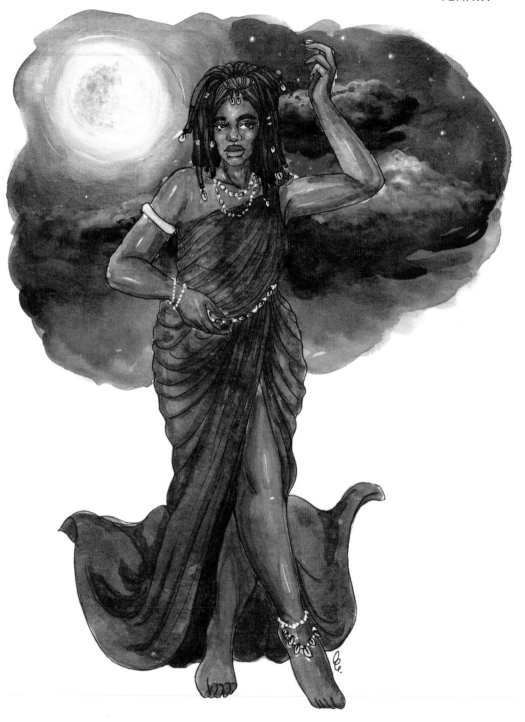

The Scorpio myth is a beautiful example of the healing and transformation that forgiveness offers. Scorpio, signified by the scorpion with pincers holding on, by the serpent shedding its old skin, or by the eagle flying high and free, is the blueprint of transformation. Forgiveness is the impetus of that transformation. We are karmically carrying all or none of the forgiveness our parents carried. Our bodies store these memories of harm from generation to generation. We can choose to release this burden by letting go and shedding the old, in our lifetime, laying down the weight of martyrdom and flying high and free like the eagle.

Forgiveness does not mean we expect to hear "sorry" from others. It has more to do with us. Sometimes forgiveness cannot be the goal, and the willingness to forgive is the aim. It's a choice to be easy on ourselves and let go and live in a spirit of release. The process of release and grieving often feels circular. Many times what I thought was released becomes triggering again. Being present to that knowing tells me I am making progress in healing. It begins with awareness and moves from that place into release.

Be gentle and compassionate with yourself as you move through this process, as you let go. Use all your tools, including plant medicine, to support this journey. Visualize release. Energy responds to the imagination. If you can see and feel what release feels like there, it becomes easier to manifest here. We can allow ourselves to transform in every given moment.

Your sexual health system has a relationship with the Moon and Yemaya; our primordial mother of creation is also the ocean's mother. This relationship demonstrates our proximity to universal energies. When the tide comes in, our bodies respond with our cycle. Many of our bodies respond to this pull by bleeding on a full Moon. The Moon's fullness is felt in our bodies and then releases stored energy, blood, our innate connection to nature.

Our lives can reflect and honor the cycles of the Moon. We can be full and also live in complete emptiness. We learn this lesson by looking at nature and knowing that we are cyclical beings like the Moon; we can be full of light or dark. At no point should we tell ourselves that we need only be one expression of our wholeness. Without expectation and explanation, we can turn inside and enter into the dark, wisdom-filled place in our body. In those profoundly reflective moments, we listen to our voices and gain the wisdom we need to sustain ourselves. Ideas seeded here need to be nourished and grown by us, outside of others' purview. It is in these times when we go inside that we face our shadow, the fear that exists in being our most authentic, powerful selves, and this requires alone time.

Sexual Health

Our sexual health is related to the health of our entire bodies. Sexual energy is not separate energy that can build in a moment. Instead it is long term and parallels the health of the body. Our body holds one source of energy, which includes our sexual health. Before we can address libido, we need to first look at a person's overall lifestyle, where their primary energy gets directed. Whatever is remaining is what we have for sex and intimacy.

The digestive system and the sexual-health system are closely connected. Taste your sexual fluids, and you can taste what you've eaten. Diet is critical for being in our best sexual health. If our digestion is not functioning well, we are not feeling our most sensual. If we are sick or digesting low-vibrational food, the first thing that suffers is our libido.

When we are not well, the body sends all its energy toward the repair of those systems. Chronic illness depletes our sexual energy. Suppose you have a cold or flu; notice how your libido declines. Our vital energy first focuses on repairing, fixing, nourishing, and taking care of other bodily issues.

Bleeding

Our Moon says a lot about what's going on in our lives. One of the most informative ways to know and understand your sexual health is to track your menses if you're a body that bleeds. Menstrual health tells us much about sexual health. How we bleed is a clear indication of our body's health. Paying attention and tracking our cycles is essential. It can be the first indicator of imbalance or illness in our sexual health system. It can inform us of cysts, tumors, cancers, and other issues.

The blood we release each month is a sacrifice. It is our most potent offering that we can make to Spirit. Our bodies will make this offering approximately every 21 to 28 days, every Moon cycle. Recognize this monthly sacrifice and pray for desires to manifest in your life or for the needed release. Moon cycles are a great opportunity to work with forgiveness practices.

When we bleed, we are most powerful. The passageway is freely and fully open to all worlds, connected to all the cosmos. Conscious bleeding asks us to recognize our vulnerability and make it a practice to protect ourselves when we are bleeding. Carrying a stone or plant of protection and wearing a red cloth around the womb are some simple ways to protect ourselves from soaking up the energies of others.

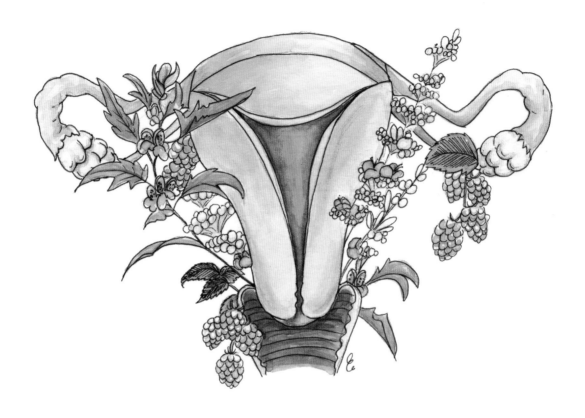

Fertility and Creativity

The ovaries are grape-sized, produce all our sex hormones, and carry 200,000 to 400,000 eggs at birth. Only 400 will release in a lifetime. Knowing this is essential when discussing fertility because our body's relationship to conception begins well before considering pregnancy.

Our body's wholeness includes fertility. Conception doesn't just happen; fertility is a magical, profoundly spiritual act. Spiritual and emotional healing often have to happen to create a fertile home for a new life.

It is through the sexual-health system that we channel our energy into our creation. Creating is life. If we do not birth physical babies, we make other things, whether it's our art form, using our voice, medicine making, drawing, singing, laughing, or dancing. All of these are creative processes. When we find ourselves disconnected from our creative processes, we disconnect from our life source, sexuality, and pleasure.

Plants for Sexual and Reproductive Health

Plants that heal the sexual and reproductive system function in an integrative way, healing body, mind, and spirit. These herbs feed the body and provide extra energy and vitality to the entire body. Some of these herbs are aphrodisiacs because they nourish the kidneys, increase stamina and desire, and enrich the libido. Simple, nourishing herbs can change a person's sexual health.

Also mentioned are plants that heal, nourish, tone, and support the womb. They help with efficient blood flow, reduce inflammation, and balance the body from puberty to menopause and beyond, nourishing us through all transitions.

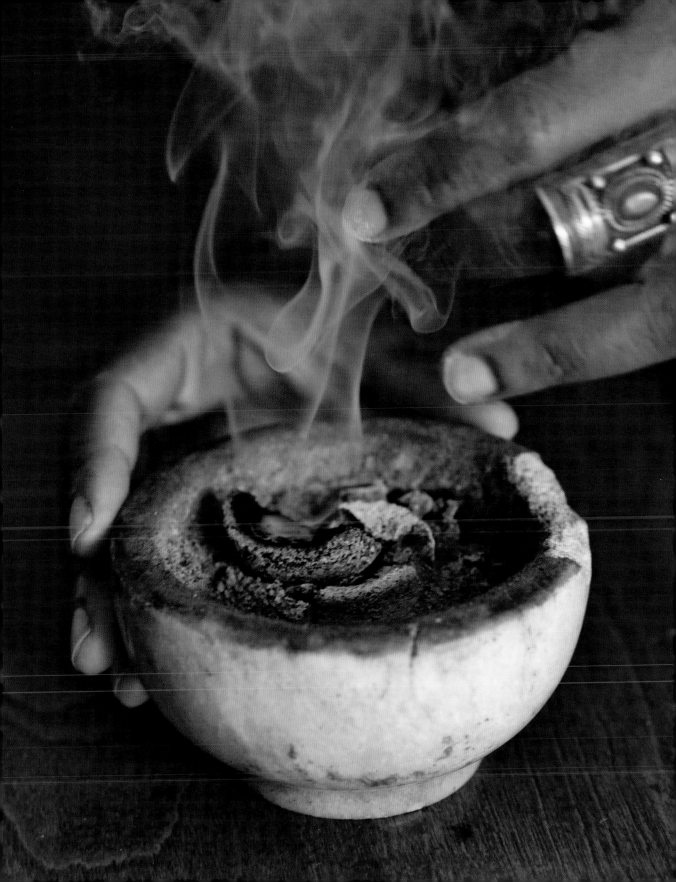

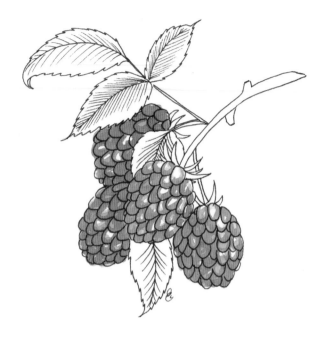

RED RASPBERRY

The epitome of self-preservation and self-love, red raspberry teaches us the efficient exchange of power and flow from fullness. It allows us to witness when we have extended ourselves beyond capacity—to give and to hold what we need for ourselves.

Red raspberry is widely known for balancing sexual health issues. It helps us maintain our strength through all transitions, and it nourishes the creative life force energy of the feminine. Rich with tannins and deeply astringent, red raspberry tightens all things that are overflowing, including how we bleed. When we bleed heavily, we are overgiving our life force. Red raspberry facilitates efficient bleeding, mentoring us in using power.

In our herbal apprenticeship program, we speak of raspberry as a power workout. As it tones and strengthens the uterus, it conveys the vital lesson of overgiving, not letting our power escape us. It protects us from giving in excess, showing us how to be in the flow of giving and receiving so we maintain control.

As with all plants in the Rosaceae family, red raspberry has thorns, reminding us that individuals should approach beauty with respect. It is protective of the feminine and can be hung in places where protection is needed.

Common Name: Red Raspberry

Latin Name: *Rubus idaeus*

Other Names: Garden Raspberry

Taxonomy: Rosaceae

Botanical Description: This bush features alternate leaves with three to seven leaflets. The green leaves have whitish undersides. Raspberry bears red fruit on thorny, arching canes.

Native Habitat: Europe; Asia

Wildcrafting and Cultivation: Gather leaves before flowering and fruiting takes place. Grow from seed; raspberry likes full sun and some afternoon shade.

Parts Used: Leaves and sometimes the fruit

Planetary Influence/Correspondence: Venus, Water

Energetic Quality: Mild, bitter, cool

Pharmacological Constituents: Tannins; flavonoids; glycosides; vitamin B; iron; manganese; magnesium; potassium; very high in vitamin C (fruit)

Ethnobotanical/Historical Use: Native Americans used raspberry in smoking rituals; People from the SWANA region fed the leaves to their stallions for sexual health.

Actions/Properties: Astringent; alterative; antiabortive; antiemetic; antispasmodic; diaphoretic; hemostatic; laxative; oxytocic (releases oxytocin from the brain—birth, sex, and pleasure hormones, triggers uterine contractions and orgasms); parturient (helps the entire birth process, especially after childbirth, helps the placenta come out); refrigerant (cools the body internally); stimulant; tonic

Indications: Plant ally for every stage of life; puberty; menstrual cramps and excessive menstruation; normalizes blood flow for young people; leukorrhea (excessive vaginal discharge); tightens and tones the uterus; uterine prolapse; used after birth to restore the uterus; diarrhea; nausea; vomiting; sore throat; canker sores; enriches breast milk; because of tannins helps with wounds and sores; conjunctivitis; mucous membrane and gums

Contraindications: People who are already cold and dry or who have chronic constipation should not use raspberry.

Methods of Preparation and Dosage

Infusion: Make a nutritive infusion by adding 1 tablespoon (2 g) dried leaves to 1 cup (235 ml) water. Steep overnight.

External Use: As a vaginal steam for uterine prolapse (see page 114).

Eyewash (for conjunctivitis): Make a strong tea and rinse your eyes.

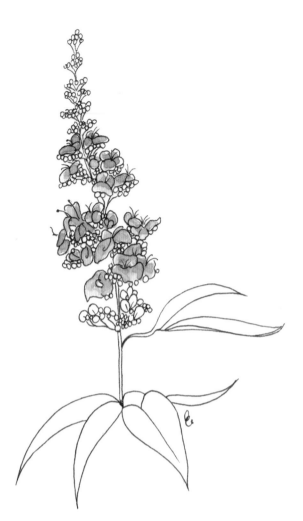

VITEX

Who is your favorite, most reliable aunt? A trustworthy, sexually alive, and independent aunt. One with whom you can be most honest about all things in your sexual life, and who gives you direct and honest advice that pulls you back into balance and then leaves you to stand in your own power.

In my apprenticeship program, that aunt would be the energy of vitex. Vitex is a graceful teacher who brings harmony to the body and spirit. It instructs in the acceptance of feminine energy and sexuality. It is both a stimulant and a relaxant. It can increase libido or decrease libido and teaches us how to moderate sexual energy. It regulates estrogen and progesterone, adjusting the body to its unique natural rhythm. And it is helpful to young people as they begin to understand the cycles of life. It shows us how to own our power as we transition through all life stages, creating intuition in our bodies, and knowing when to hold on and when to release that power.

Vitex is also called chaste tree berry and was once carried as a symbol of chastity and virginity. Vitex explores the nature of the word *virgin* to its original meaning of autonomy over the self, not needing another to be self-sufficient, and reminding us of the work of the temple priestess Ishtar, who was considered virginal despite her sex work. The nature of vitex is autonomy, ownership over our innate sexual power. It centers and stabilizes our life force energy.

Common Name: Vitex

Latin Name: *Vitex agnus-castus*

The Art & Practice of SPIRITUAL HERBALISM

Other Names: Chaste Tree, Monk's Pepper, Chaste Lamb

Taxonomy: Verbenaceae

Botanical Description: This beautiful, aromatic tree grows from 6 to 20 feet (2 to 20 m) tall; it bears spikes of lilac-colored flowers followed by small, gray fruit, with a distinct aroma.

Native Habitat: Mediterranean; Asia; cultivated everywhere

Wildcrafting and Cultivation: Gather berries when ripe; grows in well-drained, dry soil.

Parts Used: Fruit

Planetary Influence/Correspondence: Mars, Water

Energetic Quality: Bitter, acrid, warm

Pharmacological Constituents: Volatile oils; bitter principle; alkaloids; glycosides; flavonoids; iridoids (hormone balancing)

Ethnobotanical/Historical Use: Used as a reproductive tonic since the Middle Ages. The berries reduce libido in men and were given to monks to promote chastity. Virgins carried it as a symbol of their virginity in Greece and Rome.

Actions/Properties: Amphoteric (can act as an aphrodisiac or an anaphrodisiac); glandular tonic; hormone balancer and regulator; fertility enhancer; galactagogue; supports the corpus luteum (around the egg); an affinity for the second half of the cycle (PMS); works slowly and should be used for one to four menstrual cycles

Indications: PMS and all the symptoms (moody, weight gain, nausea, headaches); menopause; estrogen-dominant people who bleed too frequently, i.e., during mid-cycle; helps balance estrogen and progesterone in the body; fibrocystic breasts; libido balancer; infertility caused by low progesterone levels (often the case for infertility); coming off of birth control (to help normalize hormones); fibroids; endometriosis; teenage acne; girls who just started their periods; as a galactagogue it helps jump-start breastfeeding (use for first 10 days and then stop once milk comes in)

Contraindications: Overproduction of progesterone; deficiency of estrogen; pregnancy; breastfeeding; prepubescent children; birth control; hormone replacement therapy; medications that bind to dopamine receptors (e.g., Prozac, other antidepressants). Not for use while bleeding.

Methods of Preparation and Dosage

Vitex is a balancer and needs to be used for 3 to 4 months. I find that it is more useful in tincture than in tea.

Infusion: Crush 1 tablespoon (6 g) vitex berries and steep in 1 cup (235 ml) boiling water for 20 to 25 minutes.

Tincture: Use 60 drops once a day upon waking in the morning.

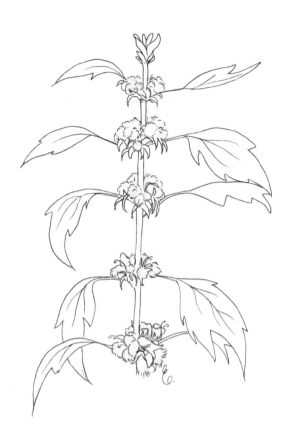

MOTHERWORT

Motherwort is one of my favorite plants to recommend when learning to mother or nurture the self. This mother's herb teaches us how to be our mothers when we did not have a model. It is excellent to restore our mothers' relationship and support the grief and loss of losing a mother. Motherwort is called lionheart, as it builds a strong and courageous heart. In my practice I call on it often to comfort a person and restore the uterus after a miscarriage or an abortion. My apprentices have called motherwort that nonjudgmental, superloving mom who holds you through all the transitions from birth to motherhood to menopause.

Motherwort has a deep connection to the uterus and the heart. From my shamanic teacher, I learned that the womb and the heart share a beat. Motherwort is the link to that beat. It connects the womb and heart and strengthens a weak heart to heal womb trauma. We cannot do womb work without addressing the heart, as traumas are stored in both the womb and the heart. This plant teaches us to flow from the heart, addressing deep-rooted ancestral trauma stored in the womb.

It brightens, soothes, and lifts the spirit, helping with heartache and heartbreak. It holds you through transitions and deepens the intuition. Motherwort is cooling and brilliant for hot conditions, such as anxiety and panic attacks. I have used it for anxiety that causes a racing heart and social anxiety.

Common Name: Motherwort

Latin Name: *Leonurus cardiaca*

Other Names: Mother's Herb, Lion Heart

The Art & Practice of SPIRITUAL HERBALISM

Taxonomy: Lamiaceae

Botanical Description: This perennial herb grows up to 5 feet (1.5 m) tall and features square, purplish stems, opposite palmate leaves that are deeply divided, and pink to purple flowers.

Native Habitat: Temperate Asia; Europe; Russia

Wildcrafting and Cultivation: Gather leaves and flower tops. Plant in rich, moist, well-drained soil.

Parts Used: Leaves and flowering tops

Planetary Influence/Correspondence: Venus, Water

Energetic Quality: Bitter, spicy, cold

Pharmacological Constituents: Iridoids; triterpenes; flavonoids; acids and alkaloids (which have a uterine stimulant effect); saponins; glycosides; tannins; essential oils; resin; calcium; trace minerals; vitamin A

Ethnobotanical/Historical Use: Chinese legend says that sages who drank motherwort daily would live to over 300 years old. Chinese courtesans would use motherwort to protect from sexually transmitted diseases. Eclectic physician Nicholas Culpepper used motherwort to dispel vapors of the heart and make the mind cheerful.

Actions/Properties: Emmenagogue; parturient; antispasmodic; cardiac tonic; hypotensive; diuretic; diaphoretic; carminative; menopausal tonic; calmative and relaxant; long-term kidney restorative; thyroid inhibitor

Indications: Heart issues associated with menopause; weak heart; suppressed or delayed menses; hot flashes; insomnia; mental and emotional stress; thyroid hyperfunction; PMS; menstrual cramps; useful to kick-start labor; aid in expelling a retained placenta; useful for midwives in birth

Contraindications: Dependence on energy modifiers, such as coffee, marijuana, sleeping pills, etc.; pregnancy; anticoagulant use; beta-blockers or cardiac glycosides; heavy menses; menopausal flooding; and hypothyroidism. Motherwort is a long-term remedy with cumulative results.

Methods of Preparation and Dosage

Fresh Tincture: Use 15 to 30 drops of tincture 3 times a day as needed.

Vinegar Extract: Add 1 teaspoon to 8 ounces (235 ml) water.

Infusion: Add 1 tablespoon (15 ml) to 1 cup (235 ml) boiling water and steep for 20 to 25 minutes. Use 3 times a day. The cold infusion is best for heart issues. Hot infusion is best for uterine issues or to increase lactation. To kick-start labor, use ½ teaspoon every half hour.

ADDITIONAL PLANTS

Mugwort *Artemisia vulgaris*

Mugwort is a rampant weed and found all over the northeastern United States. It is plentiful here in my hometown of Brooklyn, New York. I like to teach that herbs grow where they are needed. With that being the truth, mugwort's prolific growth tells us all that we need visionary dreams to move us forward in our liberation. Mugwort is a dream herb and facilitates lucid dreaming.

Mugwort's name artemisia is from the goddess Artemis, the goddess of the hunt, the Moon, and patron of women, indicating its strength and uses in feminine issues. The Moon and Water guide this plant, and the silver on the back of the leaves indicate that.

Mugwort guides us through release. It is the perfect plant for womb healing work. Take it at the end of the menstrual cycle to encourage an efficient and full flow, releasing all things stagnant. This plant is often used as vaginal steam to support healing fibroids and cysts and cervical issues (see page 114).

Contraindications: Pregnancy and nursing; heavy bleeding; extended periods

Damiana *Turnera aphrodisiaca* and *Turnera diffusa*

Damiana is a warm, spicy, and aromatic herb with a history of use as a powerful sexual tonic. Within Latin America, it was considered only second to chocolate as an aphrodisiac. I believe that the best sexual tonics or aphrodisiacs are also nervous system tonics. Damiana is just that, a nervine and a hormonal balancer.

Guided by Mars, this plant lights the sacred fire and brings warmth to a frigid and cold libido. Damiana is excellent to use for disconnection from sexual pleasure due to trauma. It teaches what it feels like to have wholeness, warmth, and feeling in our lower chakras and sexual organs.

This plant is also one of my favorite plants for dreaming, and I would never forget the dreams that damiana brings to me. Damiana dreams are watery, lucid, visionary dreams. I recommend it to people who are seeking to dream about their future lover. It can be used in a bath before bed or in a dream pillow, or in a dream tea to support your dreamwork.

Damiana centers and grounds and has a life-enhancing effect on the body and mind. Use in infusions and spells for lust. It is often drunk in liquors or cordials that are sipped slowly. Use for low libido, hot flashes, sexual exhaustion and weakness, vaginal dryness, anxiety, and depression.

Contraindications: Pregnancy; excess inflammatory conditions; long-term use can interfere with iron absorption

The Art & Practice of SPIRITUAL HERBALISM

Cinnamon *Cinnamon aromaticum*

Most of us already have this powerful medicine in our homes. Cinnamon is a digestive aid, useful for appetite loss, nausea, gas, and bloating. It balances blood sugar and curbs a sweet tooth. It enhances the digestibility of dairy and aids in the digestion of dishes that contain dairy. Use it as a tea before travel to help with is motion sickness; I have recommended that folks even carry it on their person when traveling, which does the trick. It just needs to be around you to be beneficial—a testimony to the strength of this plant. Cinnamon is helpful for those with poor circulation and for people who are always cold.

Cinnamon, guided by the Sun and Fire, is perfect for the sexual health system, requiring warm and moving herbs. It is hot and yang, meaning it moves chi, our body's energy force, promoting sexual arousal. Stuck chi often shows up as stagnation and cold. Cinnamon brings the fire! It is good medicine for those who are distant and disconnected from their emotions. It encourages love, success, and prosperity.

Cinnamon warms you up and brings passion and pleasure back to your life. Use the bark in a sensual massage oil. Add the powder to a nourishing smoothie. The bark blends well with rose and damiana in an aphrodisiac elixir. The tea of the bark blends well with rooibos and rose as a pleasurable opening tea.

Contraindications: Avoid with hot, feverish conditions with excess dryness. Avoid large amounts during pregnancy and nursing, as it decreases milk supply. Large doses can cause delirium.

Sweeten Up Yoni Steam or Bath

Yoni steams have a long history as a practice to bring wellness to the pelvic floor and sex organs and nourish the womb. Historically they have been practiced across cultures after birth to heal the perineum and cervix and tonify the womb. Steams have also been used for a prolapsed uterus, to abate infection, as a fertility practice, and to heal fibroids. Herbal baths and steams work by opening the body's tissues to receive an herb's healing components.

This yoni steam recipe I am sharing with you centers pleasure and self-care. We have used this recipe at Sacred Vibes Apothecary for more than a decade. I recommend using it following the monthly Moon cycle, and at any time you may want to center pleasure and do something lovely for yourself. We have gotten feedback over the years of the absolute pleasure using this steam has brought. Many of our customers have shared the beautiful dreams they have had after its use. I recommend using this medicine and then wrapping yourself in a blanket and heading to bed.

Many special boxes and seats are now designed for yoni steams. Purchase one if this becomes a regular practice. However I have found the recommended method works just as well.

¼ cup (8 g) dried roses

¼ cup (8 g) dried chamomile flowers

¼ cup (8 g) dried mugwort leaves

¼ cup (8 g) dried red raspberry leaves

Yield: 1 steam or bath

For a bath, mix all the ingredients in a medium-size bowl. Make a strong infusion by pouring 8 cups (1.9 L) boiling water over them. Let sit for 40 minutes. Strain the plant material using a fine-mesh sieve, discard the plant material, and add the liquid to warm bathwater.

To safely do a yoni steam, place the herbs in a pot and add hot water. Let the herbs steep for about 15 minutes. Place the pot with the herbs under a slatted chair or stool. Sit over the pot without your underwear for at least 20 minutes. To keep the steam in, wear a long skirt or wrap your lower half in a blanket. Keep your feet warm with heavy socks. Keep a safe distance between the pot and your vulva. When finished, lay quietly wrapped in a blanket and relax deeply.

Fire Starter Aphrodisiac Elixir

There is nothing better than a spicy, warm elixir to light the sexual fire. Here is a recipe I have shared with my class over the years to stimulate and bring warming to our sexual organs. It tastes delicious, and you will not have an issue convincing anyone to share it with you. Please feel confident in using it to get in touch with your pleasure.

1 tablespoon (3 g) dried damiana herb	Honey
1 tablespoon (2 g) dried roses	1 teaspoon rosewater
1 (¼-inch or 6 mm) piece cinnamon stick	Vanilla extract
1 or 2 cardamom pods	**Yield:** 6 ounces (170 ml)
6 ounces (170 ml) dark rum	

Place the damiana, roses, cinnamon, and cardamom in a clean 8-ounce (235 ml) wide-mouth mason jar. Pour the dark rum over the herbs. Add honey to taste. (Use honey to sweeten up the medicine; however, the herbs' taste should stand out, so be careful of oversweetening.)

Add the rosewater and a few drops of vanilla extract to your liking. Cap and give it a good shake. Store this medicine out of direct sunlight for 4 to 6 weeks, shaking every so often.

After that time, strain off the plants using a fine-mesh sieve. Discard the plant material. Retain the liquid, storing it in a dark dropper bottle. Use this medicine by dropping 30 to 90 drops into your mouth daily as needed.

Sacred Womb Tea

For more than a decade, we have used this tea to nourish and heal the womb. We recommend it for healing fibroids, for cysts, for use during bleeding, especially in heavy menses, after bleeding to tone the uterus, for uterine prolapse, and to prepare for conception. The tea is formulated with astringent, nourishing, and toning herbs that aid in strengthening the uterus.

1 tablespoon (3 g) dried nettle leaves

1 tablespoon (3 g) dried oatstraw

1 tablespoon (3 g) dried lady's mantle

1 tablespoon (3 g) dried red raspberry leaves

1 tablespoon (3 g) dried spearmint leaves

Yield: Enough for 4 cups (940 ml) of tea

Blend all the herbs in a bowl. For each cup of tea, use 1 tablespoon (4 g) of the herbal mixture per 1 cup (235 ml) boiling water. I recommend infusing the herbs overnight as a nutritive infusion. Drink the tea 2 to 3 times a day for best results.

Five Flower Breast Balm

The Five Flower Breast Balm is a beautiful balm that can either support self-pleasure or open us up to the power of receiving pleasure from another. Herbal salves, oils, and butters are lovely ways to encourage and engage our sense of pleasurable touch. I have found this practice to be grounding and deeply healing.

The skin is our largest organ and can absorb medicine through rich oils and butters. I have recommended this balm for regular breast/chest care, especially for those with a history of familial breast cancer. My clients have used it for fibrocystic breast healing, healing from any breast trauma, post–top surgery, and postmastectomy.

½ tablespoon hibiscus flowers

1 tablespoon (2 g) rosebuds

1 tablespoon (2 g) lavender flowers

1 tablespoon (2 g) red clover flowers

1 tablespoon (2 g) violet flowers

3 ounces (85 ml) olive oil

3 ounces (85 ml) liquid or fractionated coconut oil

½ ounce (14 g) beeswax

½ ounce (14 g) shea butter

Rose essential oil

CBD oil (optional)

Yield: Five 4-ounce (120-ml) tins

Place all of the dried plant material in an 8-ounce (235 ml) wide-mouth mason jar. Add the olive and coconut oils. Let the herbs infuse in the oils for 4 to 6 weeks in your sunniest window, shaking often.

After 6 weeks, strain the plants out of the oil using a fine-mesh sieve. Reserve the oil and discard the plant material.

In a double boiler over low heat, melt the beeswax and shea butter into the reserved infused flower oil. Take care not to overheat or burn the oil—heat just enough for the beeswax and shea butter to dissolve.

Pour quickly into five 4-ounce (120 ml) tins or small jars. To each container, add 10 drops of rose essential oil and 15 drops of CBD oil (if using). Cover and leave until hardened. Use generously over your breast or chest, solo or with a partner.

Ancestral Practice: Honoring the Moon Cycles

My work as an herbalist and plant witch has been in a deep relationship with our mother, the Moon. The healing of our sexual health organs requires an alignment with the cyclical nature of the Moon and honoring Yemaya's spirit. Each Moon cycle, we are drawn closer back to the Source and, at the same time, we are moved forward to better understand the self. Moon cycles are the key to harmonizing our internal state, our emotions, with the natural cosmic cycle. Honoring the Moon's cycles helps us tap into our subconscious, instinctive response to occurrences in our life.

In my Moon work, I have chosen to work with the lunar cycle by looking at the cycle as two halves of a whole: new moon to full Moon and waning Moon to balsamic Moon. The first half of the cycle focuses on the conception and incubation of new desires, culminating with revealing those desires to the outside world.

The second half of the cycle allows us to find meaning and extract wisdom from our experiences. It is for deepening, dying to the old, surrendering, being present to the internal process, and profound release.

I have recommended this ritual practice around the Moon for decades to my clients. I am sure it will help you resurrect, regulate, and heal your scattered parts, creating wholeness. A group of people with a shared vision can participate in this meditation together.

Under the Moon Meditation

Begin on a new Moon. Find the place in your home to directly view the Moon. If unable to find a spot that honors where the Moon is on this specific night. Prepare a tea using any of the herbs we discussed in this chapter. I like to work with mugwort or red raspberry. Whatever you choose is best for you. Create a comfortable space to sit in meditation with your tea. Burn a sweet resin such as pine or cedar to accompany your vision.

Under the light of the new Moon, begin your meditations. Take the time to focus on the question: What would you like to conceive, grow, and nourish this new Moon? You can focus on an idea, a project, or a desire. As you receive the answer, journal any emotions, words, and sentences that might arise from that question. Hold this answer to yourself. Do not share with others who are not in meditation with you. Whatever your answer is, this is your work for this Moon cycle.

As the cycle progresses with the first quarter Moon, notice how committed you remain to your vision. It is now the time to share that vision with your community and ask for support to be held accountable for the work ahead. As the Moon swells to fullness, we must center ourselves in our desires and dive deep into our unconscious. Notice the ways you may self-sabotage. As the full Moon approaches, it's time to birth and reveal our creation. It is time to listen to the feedback of our trusted community.

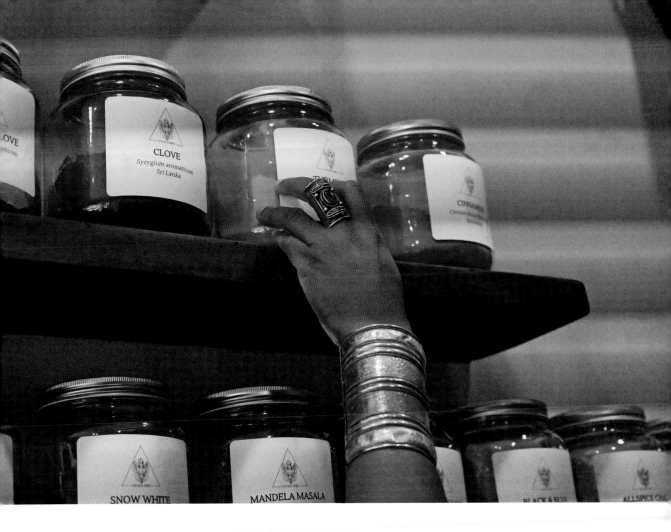

The days following the full Moon are essential to the cycle of release. We might now see what needs to change to allow this desire to come to fruition. What has reached maturity and needs to be released? Under the gaze of the full Moon, repeat the Moon Meditation at this time. Ask yourself: What needs to be confronted and released? What casted spells need breaking? And what needs transformation with love and acceptance?

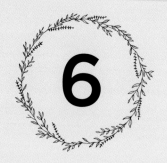

6

Healing Our Relations
SKIN HEALTH

———

Our skin, the body's largest organ, reflects our inner being. It is a revelation of the entire body's health and our relationship to the world, our families, our communities, and ourselves. On our skin, the truth does not get hidden. Our vulnerability, rage, exhaustion, and emotional capacity to deal with issues all show up on our skin.

When we have flare-ups and breakouts, it demonstrates the lack of ease and the discomfort we feel in our relationships. The sensitivity we feel on our skin speaks to our overall sensitivity. If we have cut ourselves off from the world, our skin will demonstrate our lack of ease with our environment and others. Issues such as dryness, coldness, and oversensitivity indicate our disconnection and worry. The skin becomes a mirror of whatever we are feeling inside and it responds.

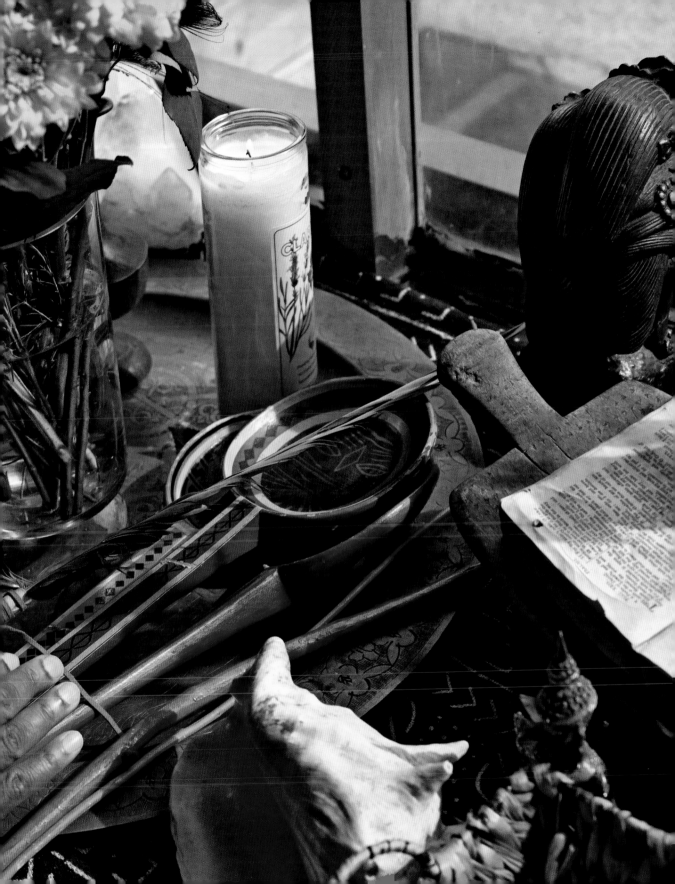

In Asian medicine, what occurs inside the body shows up through skin temperature, tone, and texture. The skin is a barometer of our body's internal health and the impact we feel from external stimuli. One way to quickly tell someone's health is to look at their skin. When things show up on our skin, it brings messages from deep inside the body to the surface for healing. The body will push any internal lack of ease to the skin's surface until we pay attention.

Our cry for help becomes public when our distress shows up on our skin, and we cannot hide the discomfort we feel anymore. We could ignore our body's unease when held in our organs, when invisible to us, but once on the skin and seeing it daily, we reach for healing. The body sends us a strong message that we can't ignore: no more hiding. This warning is a blessing, a signal that our body is still in a relationship with us, allowing us to heal our relationship with ourselves and our external relationships.

Our skin protects and alerts us. It is our external protective shield and part of the body's natural protection, the immune system. If we are feeling vulnerable and not protected, our skin and immune functions respond. When we walk into an environment that is not safe, we feel it instantly, our skin crawls, the hairs on our skin rise. It sends us a signal that we are not okay.

Our skin reflects our boundaries and ability to handle challenging situations. Have you heard folks call others thinskinned and thickskinned? We are called thinskinned because of our sensitivity. Our sensitivity is not an insult. It allows us to see, feel our emotions, have empathy, and know what situations are right for us. Living in a desensitized culture, we learn not to feel; instead, we learn to act and handle it.

When we are thickskinned, it means we have learned not to be sensitive to our environment or the people in it and to uplift our toughness. To let things bounce off of us and not be affected by what we see happening around us. We live in a world that celebrates having thick skin. Corporate environments reward those who are unbothered and deal with whatever happens. Within our current culture, we celebrate strong Black women: women who have become used to the abuse and show up and perform each day. Know that we do not have to suffer to prove that we are strong and deserving.

The Spirit of the Skin and the Relationship to Self

Your skin evokes the energy of the orisha Oshun. The most important relationship we will have is our relationship to the self, self-worth, confidence, and power. Every relationship in our life reflects the relationship we have with ourselves. One of Oshun's symbols is the mirror, the opportunity to see and appreciate beauty when we are standing in our truth; this is us in our ultimate power.

Orisha Oshun of the sweet rivers was wife to both Oggun, symbolizing strength and warriorship, and Shango, symbolizing power and kingship. Beauty and confidence are necessary to enter into a relationship with our warrior and powerful selves. The beautiful and sensual Oshun inspires us to greater harmony and acceptance of our beauty. Whenever we call her, she asks us to prioritize ourselves and our self-care. We summon Oshun to help us find our queendom. She wears a crown and sits on a golden throne; she is royalty.

Oshun is often pictured naked on top, the connection to femininity and the breasts. She asks us to honor our feminine and to understand that nurture begins with the self. It is also her encouragement for us to be vulnerable, standing bare.

When impeded with grief, fear, and anger, our organs reroute toxins to the next organ of filtration, the skin. When we are angry, we break out, inflamed and heated. This fire is the energy of Oggun. With her sweet honey, Oshun was the orisha who was able to draw out Oggun from his isolation due to anger. This legend leaves us a model to follow—to temper our anger with the sweetness of life. Honey and cinnamon are offerings to Oshun, encouraging us to open up to the sweetness life offers and be led out of our moments of sadness and isolation by connecting to joy.

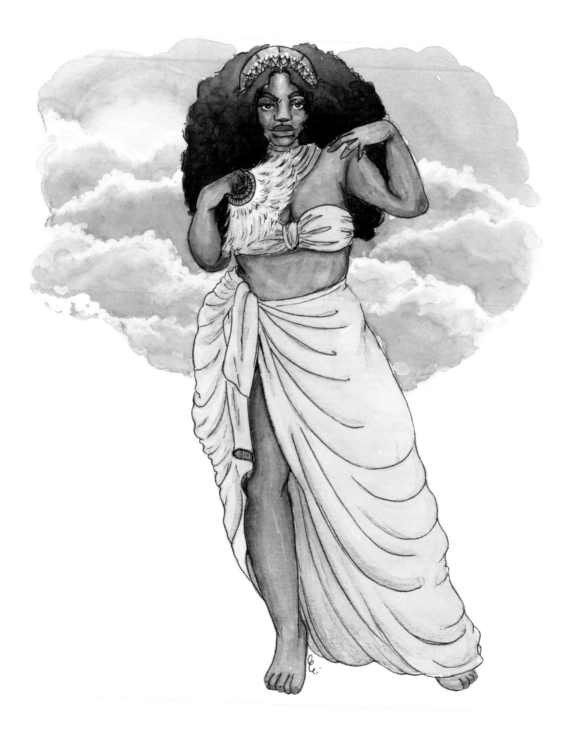

Healing Touch

The power of touch is healing and necessary. We see this demonstrated in babies who thrive when receiving skin-to-skin contact. We lose our relationship to touch when we grow up in an environment that does not encourage touch. Learning how to be comfortable with self-touch is the essential part of embracing healing touch. Where are the places on our bodies that we can begin to connect or connect further with ourselves?

Self-touch leads to a reclamation of our bodies where we can become familiar again to the pleasure of touch. We can teach people how we would like to be touched and what feels good through intimacy with the self. Heal any disconnection from traumatic experiences by leaning into the pleasure self-touch brings.

I recommend creating a beautiful skin salve to encourage this healing. A healing breast or chest salve is excellent for reconnection after top surgery, mastectomy, or breast cancer.

Healing Our Relationships
To Land and Nature

Healing ourselves from the impact of colonization and white supremacy means healing our relationship to our indigenous selves and minds. It also means healing the relationship with our homelands and the land on which we now live. Showing honor includes uplifting the people who stewarded that land and their history as land workers, farmers, healers, and caretakers. Let our movements be with sustainability in mind for a future generation every time we touch the soil.

I often hear from my students that there is a fear of being outside and being in the soil. We were taught that nature was harmful and that we would get hurt by engaging with it. Many of our parents cannot understand why we would choose to engage in herbalism and farming when they made it their business to ensure we had an education that would distance us from this legacy. For Black people, returning to farming and reclaiming our relationship with the land is a complicated relationship. We know that our ancestors did not choose to develop lands for their enslavers and that they were forced into relationships with lands far away from their homes. We realize that our bodies still live through much of that trauma. And yet, we recognize that our healing and salvation is our connection to nature and to the soil on which we live.

Research has shown that our mental health improves by being in the soil and connecting to the earth through our hands. A return to the soil has healed many of us, and it's where we feel most authentic and magical. Much of the magic we hold in our bodies requires nature as its catalyst. As herbalists, we are magicians of nature, witches, and brujas. We return to power by returning to nature. It is a direct connection to our ancestral legacy and the ultimate healer.

To Plants

As herbalists, we are plant stewards. We teach others how to heal themselves and the soil and to live relationships with plants. Each year I ask my Level II apprentices to choose a plant for a plant walk. It is remarkable to choose to be in a relationship with a plant ally. Allyship with a plant can look like spending a dedicated amount of time walking with that plant. Before this relationship begins, like any other relationship, ask the plant that shows up for you for its permission to walk with it. Any relationship we enter into should be consensual and reciprocal. The plant is an active participant, and the attraction is mutual.

Getting permission from a plant means asking and allowing ourselves to listen. Feel what happens to its leaves when you touch it and ask for permission. Does it curl around your fingertips? Does it lean into you? Does it lean away? What do you feel in your gut? Once you have received your answer, tell your plant friend what you need. And ask it what it needs from you. Spend time often with your plant friend in mediation or just sitting with it. It will teach you many things about yourself, nature, and the entire cosmology. Journal with your plant, draw your plant, make medicine with your plant.

We are protectors of our plant family as herbalists. We educate about endangered plants and protect them against threats such as overharvesting, poaching, or erratic germination rates. Make it your commitment to use plants that are local to your environment for your healing. Plants that exist in other people's environments are for their healing. We have become fascinated as a culture in utilizing exotic plants from other lands because we can. I encourage you to think of how that plant got to you. What is the chain of supply? Who planted and harvested that plant? Was it through exploitative labor? Is there any instability in local supply that our demand is seeding? Who benefits most from this plant's sale? When asking ourselves these questions, we realize that we cannot be plant and land stewards and not be involved in land justice. We often see the effect of the supply and demand chain most impacting impoverished and marginalized communities of color, which means we are engaged in racial and economic justice. Herbalism is political.

To Our Community

Who are the members of your community? Each year I give my Level II cohort an assignment. I ask them to identify the members of their community. This assignment is part of our book discussion from our required reading of *The Healing Wisdom of Africa* by Malidoma Somé. The guidelines for this assignment are to choose eight people who are our community. These individuals are determined based on their protection and unconditional love for us and how they uphold and remind us of our purpose. The responsibility of our community is to remind each other of what we came here to do. As children, we connect to our purpose, and as we grow into adults, we are programmed away from that purpose. In the indigenous community, the elders and Spirit discuss a child's purpose even before they come in. Born with their purpose, the community knows why the child has been sent and then works to uphold that purpose.

Based on this ancestral framework, I ask my students to choose their community. This exercise is often an emotional one. Some feel gratitude for the people with whom they surround themselves. Or they begin to notice how isolated they have become. Our community has not cut itself off from us; instead we have cut ourselves off from them.

Relationship building takes work. A relationship is an agreement, a contract where parties examine their needs and know what can be filled by the partnership and outline how. Any relationship between businesses, communities, or individuals stems from a need to have certain expectations fulfilled. In our culture individual relationships do not speak to their expectations and agree on what they could provide. It is common practice in indigenous culture to sit with elders in the community to outline agreements. One such example is a marriage agreement, which extends way beyond our Western marital vows. Parents, consenting individuals, and village elders outline needed requirements for all parties. They now have a working plan to move forward that outlines their agreement for their partnership.

Agreements such as these in our partnerships and friendships allow us to show up purposefully, in full authenticity, and offer room for mistakes and forgiveness. When we mess up, we see where we were out of right relationship and, if willing, we are called back to the agreement or encouraged to forge an entirely new understanding. This practice helps us move away from a culture that cancels meaningful relationships. Treasure your relationships and know that healthy familial, communal, and business partnerships are the basis for thriving communities.

To the Ancestors

Respecting and honoring the ancestors means learning who we are and who our ancestors are. The effect of colonization and white supremacy is that many of us, including white people, struggle to identify our lineage and, as a result, struggle to connect to our ancestors. Many of us have relied on DNA tracing to know our origins with some certainty. Others have taken the time to compile detailed family trees and researched ancestral lineages. For many reasons, some of us cannot trace our ancestral roots. And yet the ancestors can be connected to and honored.

Honoring our ancestors means revering them, regarding and treating them with deep respect. I am often asked how to honor ancestors we don't know. My response is to begin with one ancestor you do know. I end my conversations with my ancestors by letting them know that it was not my intention to overlook any of them. I ask to learn more about those I do not know, and ask them to step forward and let me see them in my dreams or to show up in my conversations with my family. I have met many of my ancestors this way.

Call on them often. When ready, create an altar, a meeting place for your ancestors in your home, and include their pictures and favorite things. Invite them in and let them bring life to your home. As with any relationship, building a relationship with our ancestors takes effort, perseverance, and commitment.

We can speak to our ancestors anywhere—in our bed, at our desks; they're even present in our cars. There is no particular outline for the conversations you will have with your ancestors. Conversations can look any which way, with honesty and truth. Those conversations can be sweet reunions or they can be sharing hard truths or drawing a boundary. I have learned from my mentor Thomas, a Palo and Santeria priest from Ecuadorian heritage, that those living are fully empowered. Our ancestors aren't allknowing, they are in Spirit, and we are the guides in this lifetime. We take the lead in our ancestral relationships.

I recommend telling them what is happening in our families, our communities, and our lives. It's like a phone call you would have with your grandparents, a check-in. Tell them what you need and do so often. The more you ask, the more you hold their attention.

Feed your ancestors. Light candles and offer them coffee, water, gin, rum, or any other drinks your ancestors might have enjoyed. The intention behind feeding your ancestors is to be in a reciprocal exchange. As we are requesting, we also give to their Spirits. Often when I have a big request for the ancestors, I prepare their favorite meal, not mine, and place it on the altar for their Spirits to enjoy. After removing the meal, I offer it to one of my favorite trees in the park.

Another question I am asked often is, how do we build relationships with ancestors who weren't honorable? My answer is multilayered; it includes asking why that ancestor is now calling on you to create a connection. Have they appeared in your dreams? Do you keep seeing their name? Where have you gotten the information that they were not honorable? Sometimes stories passed down in families about that difficult uncle or great-aunt speak to their relationship with that ancestor and not yours. I find these difficult uncles or great-aunts are exactly the warriors we need on the other side when it's time to call on a warrior spirit.

Other times we have ancestors we know engaged in enslavement or oppression or committed other wicked acts. This knowledge presents a need for ancestral healing. Balancing the karmic scales and working with these ancestors requires the support of your family and communities. Telling the truth, having equitable exchanges by investing your resources with the people whom your ancestors harmed in your community, and leaning on ancestral medicines make a significant difference in healing the lineage.

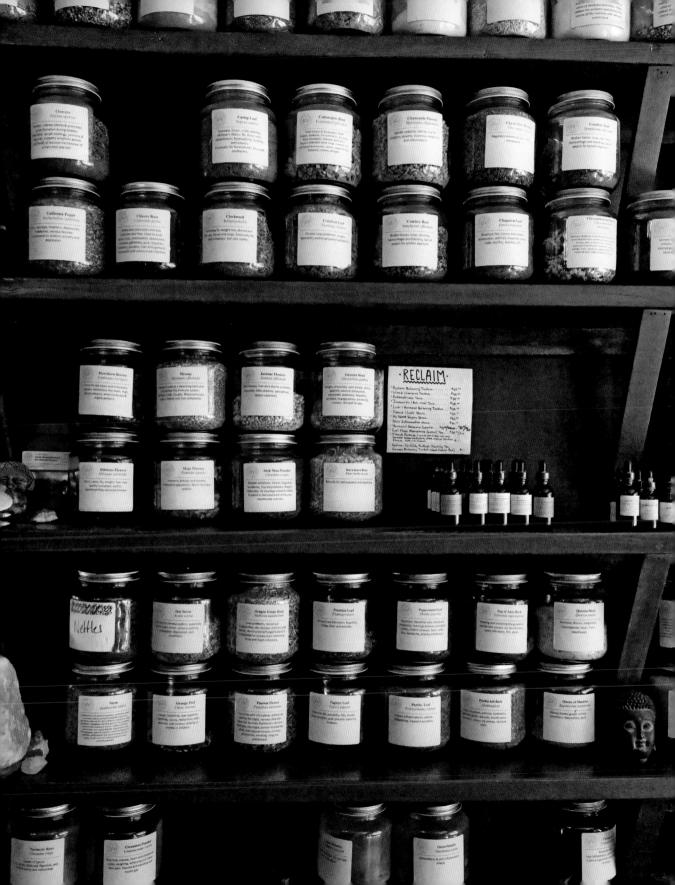

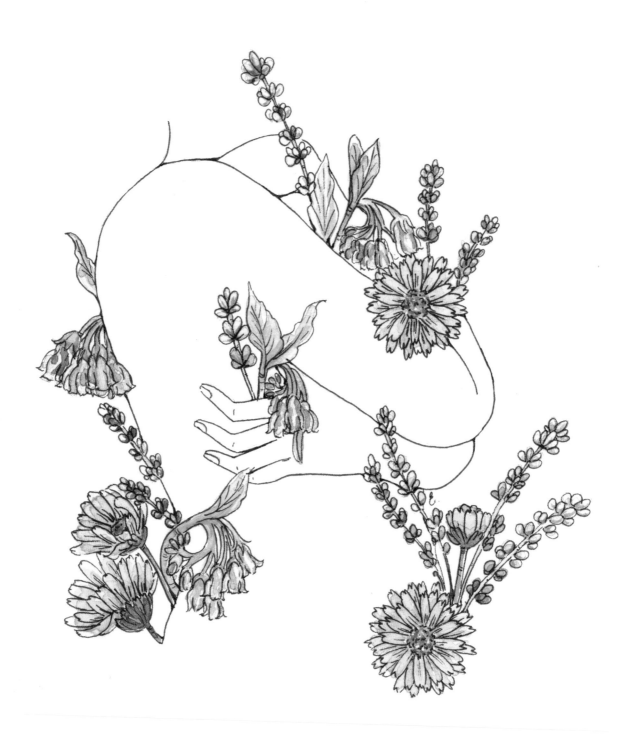

Skin Health

The skin envelopes the body with protection and keeps its temperature regulated. When exposed to heat, we sweat so that the internal organs keep the correct temperature they need for proper functioning. When it's cold outside, we shiver as our bodies try to warm up our internal temperature. In addition to regulating temperature, our skin holds in moisture and detoxifies our body by elimination.

The skin is porous and absorbs nutrients, such as water and vitamin D for the body. Whatever we apply to the skin, including all the products we use for skin care, penetrates deeply into our body and our organs. Our skin is a vital organ like our heart, lungs, and liver. If we apply products to the skin that we wouldn't eat, it is still entering our bodies through absorption. As a simple rule, if we wouldn't place it in our mouth, we shouldn't put it on the skin.

The skin is the body's largest organ of elimination. Any condition that surfaces to the skin has been progressing in the body for a while. When the skin is functioning well, it eliminates 2 pounds (907 g) of waste a day. When it is not functioning, the lymphatic system and other elimination organs—the lungs, liver, and colon—are challenged to provide this elimination. Conversely if there are issues with your lungs, liver, and colon, it shows up on your skin.

Plants for the Skin

Plants for the skin are rich in essential fatty acids, vitamin C, minerals, and potassium, and they aid in alkalizing the body and cleaning the intestines. These herbs keep our skin looking healthy and vital. To heal skin issues, we have to address blood toxicity and the eliminative organ function. The herbs recommended below heal the skin because they are blood, liver, and lymph cleansers.

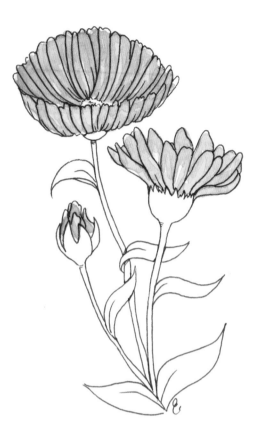

CALENDULA

Calendula, or bride of the Sun, is a beautiful plant that looks like the Sun. Its energy is yang, heating, and moving. It is both a lymphatic cleanser and a diaphoretic, opening up the skin's pores so that we can sweat. Through these actions, it helps cleanse the body of toxins that reflect on the skin. Calendula repairs and heals broken skin. It aids in building healthy granular skin tissue and reduces inflammation.

Spiritually calendula brings light to dark places, where the warmth of the Sun is needed. It renews and heals by connecting us to our joy and happiness. It is useful in times of loss or grief. It is excellent for seasonal depression, as it brings in light, warmth, and cheer. When I teach calendula, I note that healing doesn't have to be painful. Healing can come through adding more love, joy, and warmth to our lives instead of stripping things away.

Calendula helps people who speak superficially and are listening to respond and not to hear genuinely. It increases understanding and receptivity, and encourages warmth, sensitivity, and better communication. You can place calendula in a bowl where there are difficult conversations to be had.

Common Name: Calendula

Latin Name: *Calendula officinalis*

Other Names: Pot Marigold, Marigold, Maribud, Bride of the Sun

Taxonomy: Asteraceae

The Art & Practice of SPIRITUAL HERBALISM

Botanical Description: This multibranched annual has oblong leaves, a solitary ray flower that is cream to dark orange, and a distinct aroma.

Native Habitat: Central Europe; Canary Islands; Mediterranean; North Africa; Iran

Wildcrafting and Cultivation: Cultivated; plant by seed in January in a prepared bed

Parts Used: Flowers

Planetary Influence/Correspondence: Sun, Fire

Energetic Quality: Yang, spicy, bitter, neutral, cool

Pharmacological Constituents: Essential oils; saponins; resin; bitter principle; triter-penoids; flavonoids

Ethnobotanical/Historical Use: Twelfth-century sources note that calendula was used for clearing the eyesight and the head, and to encourage cheerfulness. This plant was dedicated to the Virgin Mary. It also has a history of use as a plant dye.

Actions/Properties: Anti-inflammatory; antispasmodic; astringent; vulnerary; emmena-gogue; antimicrobial; antifungal; alterative; bitter; cholagogue; diaphoretic; anthelmintic; antiviral; hemostatic; normalizes female reproductive cycle; promotes the formation of granular tissue

Indications: *Externally:* Heals and clears inflammation; rapid wound healer; rashes and warts; fungal infections; ulcers; wounds; burns; sores; diaper rash; cracked and dry skin; chickenpox; eye infections; cuts; bruises; shingles. *Internally:* Gastritis; ulcers; candida; fungal infection; delayed or irregular menses; hemorrhoids; lymph congestion; colds and flu; liver issues such as hepatitis and jaundice.

Contraindications: Do not use during early pregnancy because it is an emmenagogue. Apply calendula to clean wounds because it heals quickly and can close dirt in a wound.

Methods of Preparation and Dosage

Infusion: Add 1 tablespoon (3 g) to 8 ounces (235 ml) boiling water. Let steep for 20 to 25 minutes. Use 2 to 3 times a day.

Tincture: Use 30 to 60 drops of tincture 3 times a day.

External Applications: Use as an herbal oil, salve, cream, or lotion.

Bath: Use calendula as a vaginal steam (see page 114) or as a sitz bath for hemorrhoids.

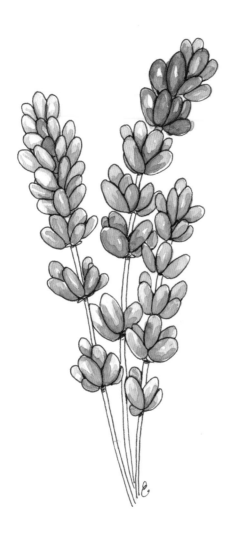

LAVENDER

Aromatic lavender gets its name from the word Latin word *lavere*, which means "to wash." Many cultures have used lavender to bring a lovely aroma into their home. Delicate yet powerful, lavender can heal staph and strep, systemic infections, and many viruses. Old herbal books state that prostitutes wore lavender to advertise their profession. I believe that lavender was worn and used as protection, as it helps to heal many sexually transmitted diseases. It helps us stand in our choices and be protected.

Guided by Mercury, lavender lives in duality all the time and encourages us to do the same. It is amphoteric, an herb that can be both a stimulant and a sedative. It stimulates digestive organs, aids with digestion, and uplifts the mood. Simultaneously it relaxes and sedates the nerves and benefits anxiety, PMS symptoms, and menopausal symptoms.

One of my apprentices once called lavender a "mother of dragons." We see this clearly in how lavender combines softness and fierceness. Lavender is a fierce protector and somewhat of an unexpected warrior. It is excellent for working through fear. It is said to help us see ghosts at night, holograms of our fear. It allows us to see our fears and conquer them.

Lavender's protective and calming energy acts on thoughts and protects from repetitive negativity and harsh self-criticism. It teaches self-love and brings peace. It is a favorite of mine for clarity and purification. Use it in baths to open the third eye to spiritual connection, providing clarity of sight.

Common Name: Lavender

Latin Name: *Lavandula angustifolia*

Other Names: Elf Lead

Taxonomy: Lamiaceae

Botanical Description: This small, tender shrub grows 1 to 4 feet (30 to 122 cm) tall; it is covered in grayish down, the leaves are opposite and narrow, and the aromatic purple flowers grow in spikes.

Native Habitat: Mediterranean region; naturalized everywhere

Wildcrafting and Cultivation: Cultivated by seed in dry soil; full sun

Parts Used: Flowers

Planetary Influence/Correspondence: Sun, Mercury, Air

Energetic Quality: Cool, dry, yang

Pharmacological Constituents: Flavonoids; essential oils; tannins; coumarin; triterpenoids

Ethnobotanical/Historical Use: Before World War I, lavender was used as an antiseptic to dress wounds. In the Middle Ages, lavender flowers were strewn across floors to release their aroma when stepped on and to repel moths. Women who wore corsets used lavender to wake when they fainted. During the plague, lavender was burned in sickrooms to help prevent the spread of disease.

Actions/Properties: Analgesic; anaphrodisiac; antibacterial; antidepressant; antifungal; anti-inflammatory; antiseptic; antispasmodic; aromatic; bitter; carminative; digestive; expectorant; nervine; rubefacient; sedative; stimulant; tonic; amphoteric

Indications: Clears heat; calms nerves; settles digestion; good for asthma when connected to anxiety; colic; fainting; dizziness; depression; fear; halitosis; insomnia; hypertension; irritability; muscle spasms; pain; stress; nervousness; wound healing; typhoid; staph; strep; diphtheria; flu; viruses

Contraindications: Do not use lavender in large doses during pregnancy.

Methods of Preparation and Dosage

Infusion: Add 1 teaspoon dried lavender to 1 cup (235 ml) boiling water. Steep for 10 minutes. Use 3 times a day.

Tincture: Use 15 to 30 drops of tincture 3 times a day or as needed.

External Use: Use a strong infusion of 1 tablespoon (3 g) to 1 cup (235 ml) water. Steep for 40 minutes. Use lavender as a mouthwash for bad breath or as a douche or sitz bath for bacterial vaginosis or UTI. Use as a hair rinse for scalp health and a bath for irritable babies. Lavender oil diluted in a carrier oil can be used as a natural insect repellent and to treat insect bites. Prepare as an herbal oil for painful joints and sore muscles, and to treat cellulite.

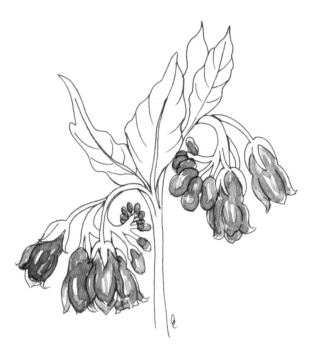

COMFREY

Knitbone, woundwort, bruisewort, and miracle herb—comfrey lives up to its name given by cultures who have used this plant for eons before us since 400 BCE. This plant's correspondence is Saturn and Water. It provides form while allowing for movement. Comfrey's energy is yin and rich in mucilage, and it deeply nourishes the body's connective tissues, hair, teeth, and skin. It is rich in allantoin, a chemical that regenerates cells. Comfrey soothes, repairs, and protects damaged tissues. Comfrey intelligence can set a broken bone when applied externally.

Comfrey rapidly brings together a fracture or a wound. This plant heals brokenness and fractures, bringing things together. It is a beautiful herb to work with to heal broken relationships, including broken relationships in your community. It is a weaver of community.

One of its contraindications is to use only if a wound is clean because of its ability to heal quickly, sealing in dirt and bacteria. I understand this to mean when the wounding is deep in our relationships, we should first clean it with the truth, an excavation of why the wounding occurred, and then use comfrey to bring things together.

Comfrey holds you together during a crisis and brings you together when you are feeling scattered. It heals a fractured spirit and helps in soul retrievals to find and integrate all parts of the soul upon return. It is binding and keeps the soul tied to the body during both astral and physical travel, as it protects against death and displacement. Comfrey has been deemed a sacred herb and is carried in a red cloth.

The Art & Practice of SPIRITUAL HERBALISM

Common Name: Comfrey

Latin Name: *Symphytum officinale*

Other Names: Knitbone, Woundwort, Bruise-wort, Miracle Herb, Gum Plant

Taxonomy: Boraginaceae

Botanical Description: Comfrey is a stout, bristle-haired perennial with thick taproots that are mucilaginous; large, tapering leaves; and bell-shaped blue to purple flowers.

Native Habitat: Europe; West Asia

Wildcrafting and Cultivation: Harvest the leaves before it flowers; gather roots in spring or fall. Grow by seed or root division and plant in partial sun.

Parts Used: Leaves, roots

Planetary Influence/Correspondence: Saturn, Water

Energetic Quality: Bitter, sweet, cool, yin

Pharmacological Constituents: Allantoin (biogenetic stimulator used to treat dry, wrinkled skin); mucilage; tannins; saponins; amino acids; minerals; pyrrolizidine alkaloids; phenolic acid

Ethnobotanical/Historical Use: Written accounts date usage back to 400 BCE. Armies of Alexander the Great used comfrey to treat wounds and bone fractures on the battlefields. Powerfully regenerative, comfrey was once given to women before marriage to restore their hymens.

Actions/Properties: Vulnerary; emollient; demulcent; astringent; anticatarrhal; antitussive; cellular proliferation; anti-inflammatory; nutritive

Indications: Soothes and protects damaged tissue; cough; wounds; sores; ulcers (internal and external); fractured and broken bones; sprains; respiratory problems; internal hemorrhages; reduces pain in bones and tendons

Contraindications: Comfrey heals wounds rapidly. The wound needs to be clean before applying comfrey. It is not suitable for deep wounds at first, as it seals the skin quickly and can trap bacteria deep inside. Do not use comfrey with liver or gall-bladder disease.

Methods of Preparation and Dosage

Infusion of the Leaves: Use 1 tablespoon (3 g) leaves to 1 cup (235 ml) boiling water. Steep for 20 to 25 minutes and use 3 times a day.

Decoction of Root: Simmer 1 tablespoon (3 g) roots in 2 cups (475 ml) water for 20 to 25 minutes. Strain and drink 3 times a day.

Tincture: Use 15 to 30 drops of tincture 3 times a day.

External Use: Use comfrey in lotions, oils, and ointments for scars, bruises, eczema, wrinkles, splinters, infections, and broken bones (splint bone first). Use in a bath to soothe and calm the skin.

ADDITIONAL PLANTS

Plantain *Plantago lanceolata* and *Plantago major*

Plantain is one of my favorite summertime herbs. Most of my summer medicine uses plantain as a base. My Rescue Balm, which I carry in my purse at all times, contains plantain, along with other helpful first aid herbs. Exposed skin in the summertime can mean bumps, bruises, cuts, scrapes, and insect bites. Plantain is a goto for addressing all these concerns. It is cooling and immediately addresses inflammation and soothes the skin. If I am without my balm, I look for a fresh patch of plantain, which grows wild throughout New York City, pick a leaf, rub it between my fingers to break the cell walls, releasing its healing components, and place the leaf on any skin irritation.

Plantain is soothing and rich in mucilage, benefiting irritated mucous membranes. It helps treat ringworm, wounds and rashes, vaginitis, urinary tract infections, and chronic coughs.

Plantain is not native to the United States. Its common names are Englishman's foot or white man's foot because it was brought here by early European colonizers in their trouser cuffs. I recommend this softening and nourishing plant often to heal the relationship white people have with their ancestors and ancestral lands.

Contraindications: Do not use in cases of profuse respiratory congestion.

Chickweed *Stellaria media*

This plant is known as starweed, as in being from the stars. Each time I see chickweed's tiny star-shaped white flowers, I think of the cosmos. Chickweed is said to allow us to be more permeable to cosmic messages. Guided by Yemaya and Water, its energy is soft and opening, and it reminds us that not all spiritual openings have to be harsh.

Chickweed opens up cell membranes so they are more porous to receive medicine and food. This healing plant is suitable for conditions that stem from excessive heat in the body, such as ulcers in the gastrointestinal tract, constipation, fever, and congestion. Externally, it helps with boils, itchy skin, rashes, eczema, poison ivy, diaper rash, and hives. Many cultures use chickweed as food and medicine. It can be picked in the early springtime and added to salads and fresh juices.

Contraindications: Do not use chickweed when there are excessive amounts of mucus in the body or during pregnancy.

The Art & Practice of SPIRITUAL HERBALISM

Violet *Viola odorata*

The joy that comes from being in violet's presence is noticeable. It is hard not to notice violet with its deep royal purple flowers. The plant's leaves are heart-shaped and are a doctrine for its work as a heart healer. Violet soothes the spirit and brings forth happiness. As a plant guided by Oshun/ Venus, it is useful spiritually to see one's innate beauty. It teaches unconditional love and opens us to connecting to joy.

It softens a hardened heart or other places in the body affected by unexpressed anger. It is useful for cysts and tumors throughout the body, especially the breast and chest, which sit over the heart. Violet helps dissolve the anger associated with overnurturing or giving in sacrifice and not from the heart.

Violet is said to have an association with the Fairy Kingdom and is useful for shy spirits. I have used this plant to encourage introverted and sensitive people to take up more space and stand in their power.

Use this plant for chronic skin conditions, rashes, psoriasis, eczema, itchy scaly skin, and skin infections. It is an excellent medicine for swollen lymph glands, urinary tract infections, and dry respiratory and digestive tract conditions.

Contraindications: Large doses may cause gastrointestinal upset and blood pressure irregularities.

Aloe *Aloe vulgaris* and *Aloe mexicana*

Every home needs an aloe plant! Many of us grew up with aloe growing in our kitchen or yards. In Sanskrit, aloe's name *kumari* means virgin or goddess, which indicates the renewing and regenerative power of this plant. Aloe can build resilience for those burned out. It helps those with creative and fiery constitutions managing their fire.

Aloe, also known as a Medicine Plant, is rich in healing and an essential first aid medicine. It is useful for skin issues such as wrinkles, burns, bruises, splinters, wounds, and diabetes foot sores. I have also used it for digestive problems such as gastric ulcers, constipation, intestinal parasites, and pinworms.

Contraindications: Pregnancy and lactation taken internally; fungal infections; externally after surgical wounds or deep wounds; bowel obstruction; GI inflammation; liver disease; kidney disease

Face Steam

One of my favorite self-care routines is face steaming. It is usually done on Mondays when my daughter Lauren spends the day with me. It is our mother-daughter bonding activity. I love steaming my face because it allows me to sit in front of a mirror for an extended time, look at, notice, and care for my face. It honors such a deep part of the psyche to notice all your facial features. I encourage you to practice this facial routine in front of a brightly lit mirror.

This steam I am sharing with you will nourish dry winter-worn skin and provide suppleness and joy! Use equal amounts of dried or fresh plants to make this steam.

2 tablespoons (4 g) dried calendula blossoms

2 tablespoons (4 g) dried violet blossoms or leaves

1 tablespoon (2 g) dried comfrey leaf

1 tablespoon (2 g) dried plantain leaf

Yield: 1 steam

Place all the herbs in a beautiful glass bowl. Boil 4 cups (940 ml) of water and pour over the flowers and leaves. Tent your head with a clean towel and sit for 10 minutes at a time, steaming your face. Take a break and steam some more. You might need to add more hot water. When finished, wash your face with cool water or follow up with a face scrub.

Rose Face Mask

Rose is especially dear to me, as it is my namesake. I use this plant of Oshun every chance I get to remind myself of my beauty and ancestral lineage. I am sharing this recipe with you as it is one of my favorite recipes to give as gifts. It is beautiful to create and is excellent to tighten and tone the skin. Making a rose mask is easy and a great way to spend an afternoon pampering yourself.

This recipe requires rose powder. You can purchase rose powder or grind it yourself in a clean and dry coffee grinder using dried roses.

¼ cup (30 g) rose powder

8–10 tablespoons (120–150 ml) rosewater

1 tablespoon (15 ml) olive or jojoba oil

Yield: 1 face mask

Place the rose powder in a clean glass bowl. Stir in the oil and rosewater until it mixes into a thick paste and turns deep burgundy. Slather the rose paste over your face, neck, and chest area, letting it dry and tighten. Wash off thoroughly, pat dry, and apply a soothing oil to the skin.

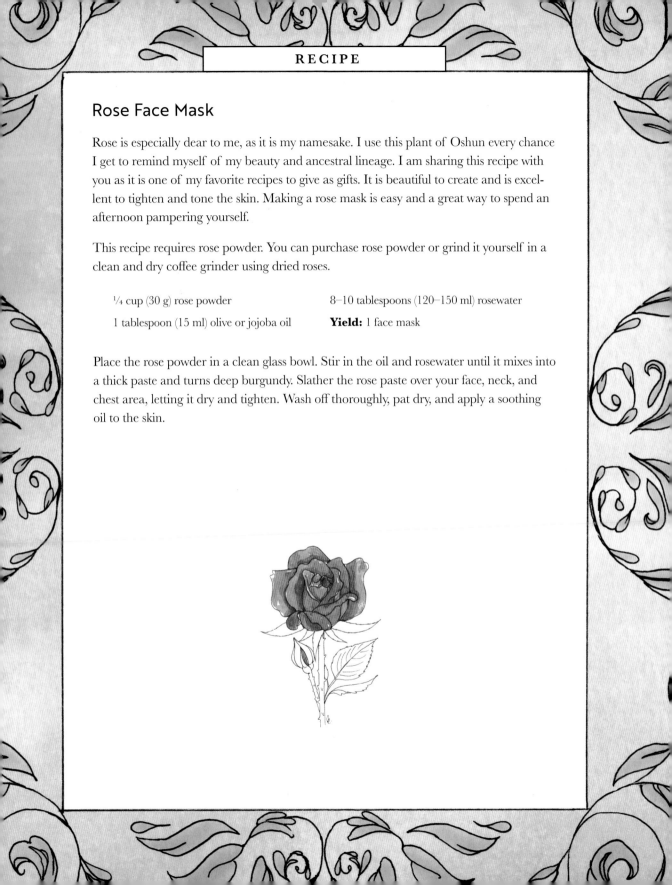

Rose Face Toner

I create my rose toner once a year with the first roses in bloom in my parents' garden. In the early summer I visit their backyard garden to harvest roses from their beautiful rosebush. The roses are a deep red, almost fuchsia. I return home carrying my precious harvest to make this face toner that lasts me all year until the next harvest. It is a profound reminder of my parents' love for me and how I can reflect that love.

I recommend making this recipe with fresh plant material. You can also substitute with dried roses. I love the beautiful pink color that results from using deep red fresh rose petals.

2 handfuls fresh rose petals

6 ounces (170 ml) pure witch hazel liquid

1 ounce (28 ml) aloe vera liquid

1 ounce (28 ml) rosewater

Yield: 8 ounces (235 ml)

Place the roses into a clean 8-ounce (235 ml) wide-mouth mason jar. Fill the jar almost full with the witch hazel. Add the aloe vera liquid and rosewater and shake very well. Cover, and label with the date, herbs, and other ingredients. Set it in a cool, dark place for 4 to 6 weeks. Shake your medicine each time you see it.

After the roses infuse into the liquid, strain off the plant material using a fine-mesh sieve. Discard the plant material and store the liquid toner in two 4-ounce (120 ml) spray bottles. I like to keep them refrigerated. It is a treat to spray your clean face with a chilled toner, especially in the summertime. This toner has an approximate 1-year shelf life.

Ancestral Practice: In My Skin: A Mirror Work Meditation

Who are we at our most essential self? The self that Spirit and the ancestors seeded? Who were we before our birth families, our educators, lovers, and employers influenced us? This mirror work practice draws us closer to who we are without the layers of expectations placed upon us.

Mirror work is a magical and spiritual practice used in many cultures. The mirror's magic is strong and ancient, and the line between this world and the other narrows on the mirror's surface.

Oshun, referred to as the Queen of Witches, is often seen with a mirror in hand, signaling that a mirror is a witchcraft tool that shows our true nature. A mirror is brilliant when working with our shadows, as it reveals the beliefs that govern our lives.

The mirror can reveal the ancestors and the rich lineage at our back and reflected on our faces. As we encounter our ancestors, it evokes remembrance and invokes their Spirits, and we receive messages and nourishment from the otherworld. This ancestral knowing is our legacy, which we alchemize into our value and worth.

Mirror Work

I love doing this magical work with a mirror that my ancestors used. If you are so fortunate to have a mirror that your ancestors used, please use that for this work. If not, I collect many vintage mirrors and cleanse them for this purpose. I especially like beautiful ornate mirrors to reflect my beauty.

This mirror work practice requires a 14-day commitment. The purpose of this practice is to see yourself in your fullness and authenticity. This practice builds a relationship with the self and with your ancestors.

Mirror work requires vulnerability, openness, and feeling safe. I usually begin with a prayer while lighting a candle to call in protective energies. At first this practice can be a difficult one, so do it when you are ready. As the days go by, I have found it becomes a meditation and even pleasurable.

You will need

• A pillow for your head or a comfortable seat

• A timer

• A yellow candle

• A mirror of your choice

• A writing instrument

• A journal

Begin by dedicating 5 undisturbed minutes of your day to your mirror work practice. Each day add a minute. On day one you will spend 5 minutes in practice. On day two you will spend 6 minutes looking at your reflection, working your way up to a full 18 minutes on your fourteenth day.

Days 1 to 7

Find a comfortable place to lie or sit. It can be in front of your ancestral altar or even in your bed.

Set your timer. Light your candle and call in your ancestors and guides to hold you in a protective space during the exercise. Relax.

Hold your mirror of choice up to your face and breathe deeply. Take three deep breaths. Settle your breathing and look at your face.

Take in your entire face without judgment. Look at yourself as a toddler would: Notice without judging, just noticing.

Notice what you are feeling. Be aware of your body, and notice where you feel tense and where you feel light. This practice is not an easy one, so take your time and be honest.

Soften your gaze and be easy with the person who is staring back at you. Notice the lines on and the structure of your face. Notice your eyes and the shape and the color, the light in them.

Continue in observation until your timer goes off. With the mirror still in hand, look into your eyes and offer words of thanks and gratitude, praising and blessing yourself for your beauty and courage.

How do you feel? Write down your feelings and observations.

Days 8 to 14

Prepare the same way as days one to seven, and on day eight, invite an ancestor that honors you to join you in your mirror. Ask them to reveal themself in your face. Who do you see?

Make the same request each day after, either asking for the same ancestor or any additional ancestors who you hold in high regard or whom you might have already built a relationship with to join you.

Spend time noticing the merge between you and your ancestors. Ask them to let you know any messages they have for you.

Continue to look at your face until the timer goes off. With the mirror still in hand, look into your eyes and offer words of thanks and gratitude to yourself and to the ancestors who joined you.

How do you feel? Write down in your journal your feelings and observations.

The Art & Practice of SPIRITUAL HERBALISM

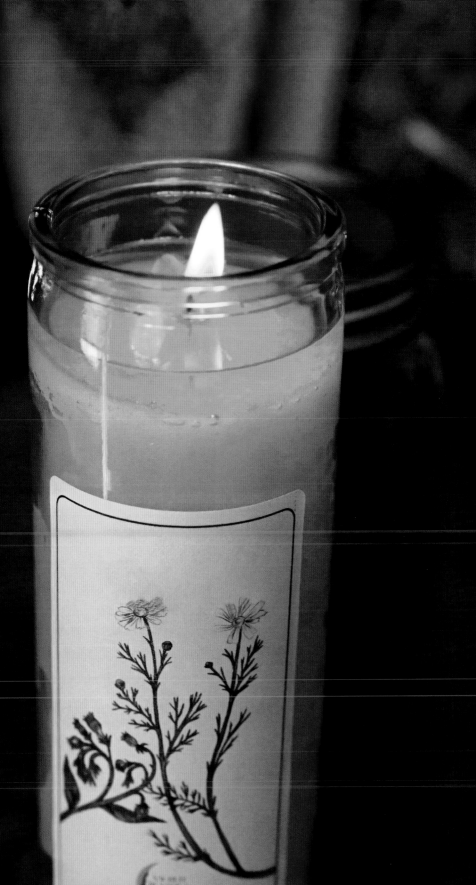

7

Listening to Spirits
NERVOUS SYSTEM

———

How does Spirit speak to you? How do you hear Spirit in your body? In what ways do you receive spiritual messages?

Whatever our Source is, any guidance we receive from Source comes through our nervous system. If our nervous system is not cared for and functioning correctly, we are not getting our messages from Spirit. We can receive messages in many forms, including through hearing, vision, colors, images, intuition, wind, physical changes in the body, symbology in the environment, synchronicities, dreams, and movement in the room. I have also heard that individuals feel Spirit when they are relaxed, have a clear mind, and feel connected and embodied, heightening their senses.

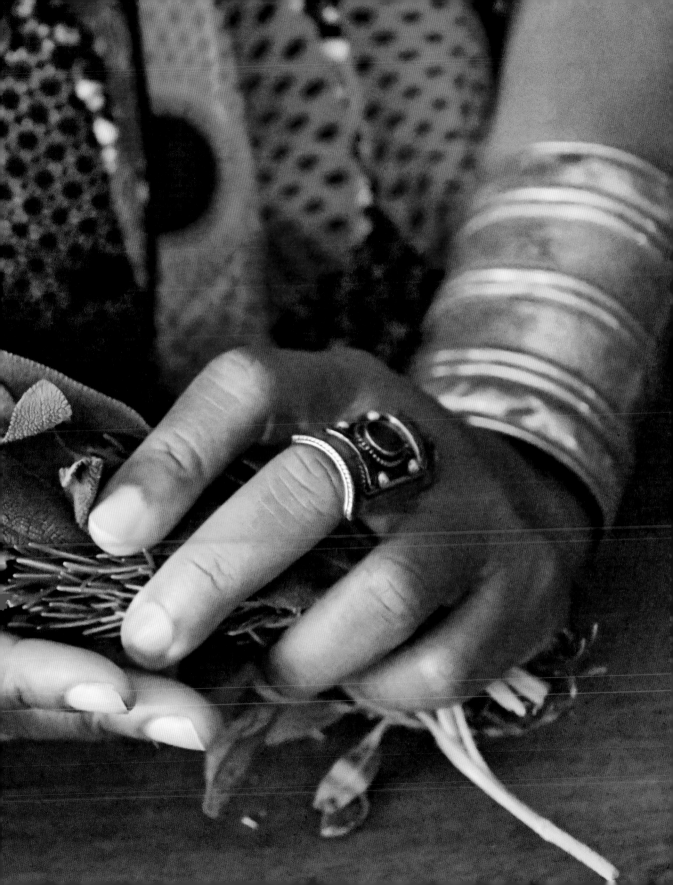

The Spirit of the Nervous System

Inspiration means when Spirit comes and fills you. We are universal beings, and when Spirit comes in, we receive messages from all things and places, past and present, back and forth, future and previous generations. These messages inspire us to create change and encourage us to take the next step in our development.

Our bodies are a vessel to connect to Spirit. Receiving messages from Spirit is an automatic download. The nervous system channels inspired messages through our senses. Often when people lack nervous system support, they experience stress. Dealing with past trauma, lack of resources, capitalism, microaggressions, and daily living demands also cause stress. This stress leaves us out of touch with the messages intended for us.

In extreme nervous exhaustion stages, we may hear many things and can't decipher where they are coming from. If we have a nervous system in crisis, we will not get our messages from Source. If we can't get messages from Spirit, we have to get information elsewhere; our messages then come only from what's in front of us—what we see, books, media, and the people in our lives—and what we receive are often illusions. Without a connection to Spirit, we lack a clear vision to discover our purpose and creativity.

We often believe that we need a healer or guru to set us straight. There is no reader or seer out there who can see better than we can for ourselves, if we are spiritually connected.

The nervous system is about connection, electricity, and messages guided by Uranus or the goddess Oya in the African diaspora. There is always the goddess of thunder or lightning and storms; this is Oya. Oya is the goddess who symbolizes our nervous system, the system of lightning and electricity. She is often called the Great Awakener. She shakes you up and asks you to be entirely part of the world you are in.

Your nervous system becomes heightened when Oya speaks. It feels like an awakening, a nervous breakdown, or a midlife crisis. Astrologers call this a Uranus transit. Indigenous cultures call this an initiation. Choosing to call this time of our lives a breakdown or a crisis is very harmful and reflects the stigma of swift and sweeping change. Even within our healing culture, we diagnose mental illness before we understand what is going on with the person and without thought to what could be happening spiritually.

Uranus or Oya's job is to change our status quo. It does not want us to continue the path we are on. When there are storms in our life, Uranus wants us to ask ourselves what entrenched belief system we must let go of—now. This urging moves us forward to a radically different framework so that we can grow.

Uranus/Oya ensures that we remain true to ourselves at the highest level. We come into this life knowing what we want, and then we get layered by experiences, childhood trauma,

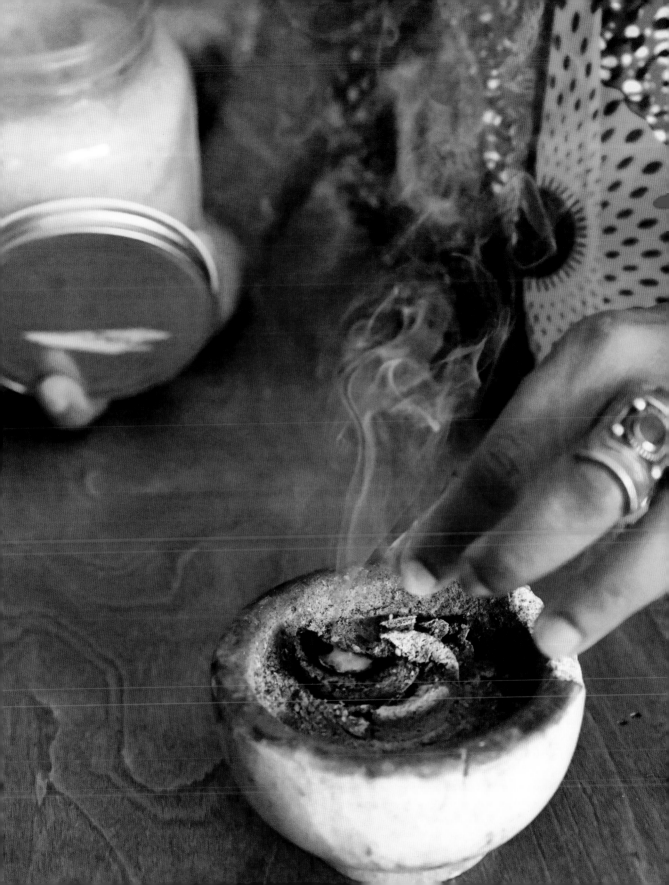

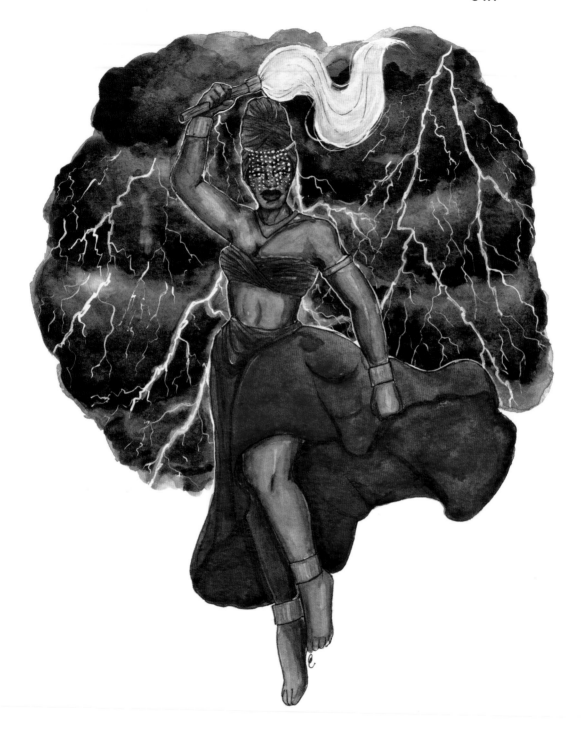

familial relationships, and partnerships. The most significant layer is fear. Our nervous system knows when we are fearful. When fear pushes up against change, it creates anxiety. Anxiety signals that we hold on tightly to an aspect of our reality that we know needs changing. When this happens, our nervous system needs to be supported to release fear to take the next step forward.

If we are alone, without a community we trust, when these transits present themselves, we could be hospitalized for a stressful crisis or breakdown when, in fact, we might be experiencing extraordinary gifts, a spiritual awakening. It is vital to have a community that can see and can name what is happening to us at this moment. The awakening comes like a bolt of lightning. It is the Tower card in the tarot deck, where everything changes overnight.

We all will face a Uranus transit in our lifetime. It is a simultaneous awakening and a release. For many of us, these intense experiences require us to revamp our lives. If we ignore the urges of this awakening, the storms will only become louder. More souls are deciding they can't deal with these awakenings and checking out in different ways. They may disassociate from their awareness and lose their minds. They may use substances, become ill, or perpetually live in crisis without making changes to alter it.

Stress and the Nervous System

When our bodies adapt to a constant state of stress, it becomes hard to recognize actual threats or danger. We may find a way to tolerate an intolerable situation by coping. The Western concept of coping becomes a way we tell ourselves that a situation is okay and live with it. It is not an indigenous concept to cope. We either leave the situation or don't. Coping is how we convince ourselves to stay in a situation we have outlived. That is one way our bodies can choose to deal with stress. We can also decide to intellectualize the pressure we are under or decide to change the situation completely.

Denial is another mechanism to deal with stress. Denial works. Denial is the partner that watches the other one smoke and get cancer. It is the person who is taking on the secondhand smoke that experiences the damage; they may not be smoking, but they are present, physically partaking in whatever is in their environment. The same thing happens to us with secondhand stress. Secondhand stress is secondary trauma. This is something that I often see happen in our close relationships.

In our relationships with the broader community, we may encounter this denial as well. Activists and healers often suffer because they continually strive to wake up individuals who are content living in a system of denial. Oppression is rooted in a system of denial. We have to activate for ourselves, and we also have to do the work of waking up others.

Ancestors and Community

Our ancestry is both spiritual and physical. There are messages left in our bodies for us: the color of our eyes, the womb shaped differently, the times we are most fertile. We are a walking, breathing connection to our ancestors, whether we acknowledge it or not. Previous experiences, our memories, and what has been coded from our ancestors also help us deal with stress. Descendants of enslaved people are gifted with resilience in their DNA, enabling their bodies to deal with some of the pressures they experience.

Past traumatic events can affect how we deal with trauma today. Encoded into our DNA are memories of stressful times. These memories and experiences stay with us and translate to how we handle situations later in life. Suppose you were poor or houseless before and then faced poverty and being houseless again. You may have developed processing and resilience methods that someone new to this exact situation may not. Stress affects everyone individually.

Support systems are an essential factor in how we handle stress. Suppose we have a community and support systems where we can share about what occurred in our day. There we will have a different response to stress than someone in social isolation who is disconnected from their community and has to process everything that happens alone. In addition to friends, family, and professional therapists and healers, we can turn to our ancestors as part of our support network.

Our ancestors are waiting for us to acknowledge this connection. Connecting to our ancestors is as simple as speaking with them. Speak with them and reach out to them. Lean on them for support and tell them all the recent happenings or challenges in your life.

The Nervous System

The nervous system is a complex electrical system connecting and transmitting information and stimuli around the body. It is also the complex electrical system that connects you to Spirit. A healthy nervous system means you can tap into messages beyond the self and deeply trust the signals received from your senses. In this era of sensory overload and constant stress, our nervous systems are more taxed than ever. In addition to delivering and receiving messages, our nervous system is home to memories, both in the brain and at the cellular level.

The brain's amygdala, our brain's memory bank, stores everything we have learned or experienced. We build up memories of touch, taste, emotion, and sound. Childhood memories are also stored and triggered by touch, smell, and taste. We can remember the taste of our grandmother's cooking during the holidays and everything about that specific day, though it was years back. We'll even remember the kitchen, the color of the walls, and the dishes on the dining table.

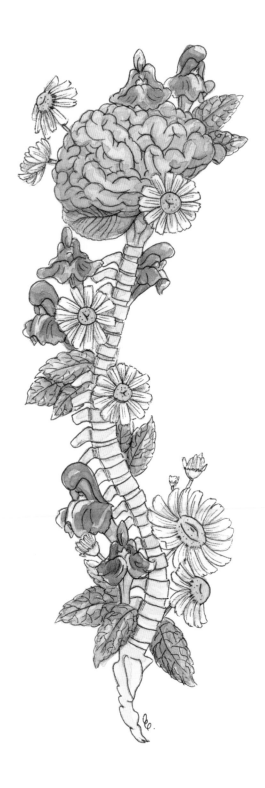

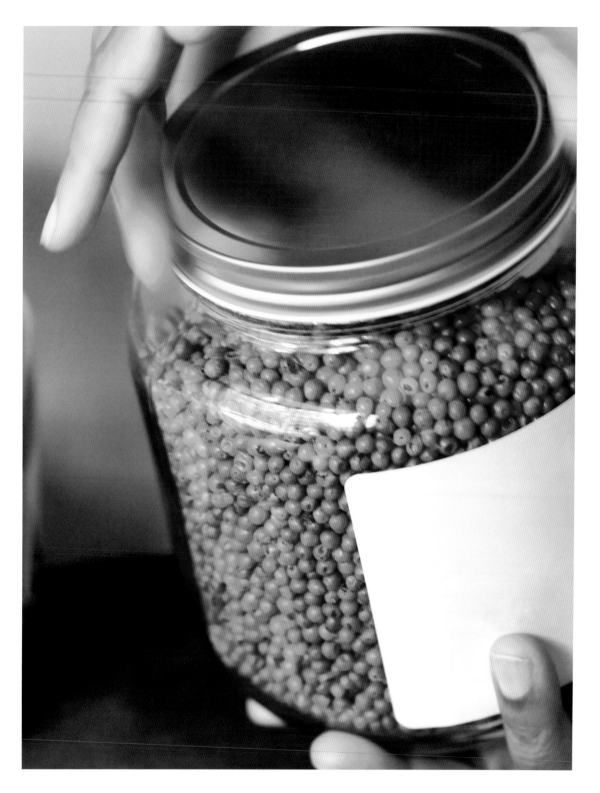

The Art & Practice of SPIRITUAL HERBALISM

The nervous system maintains homeostasis in the body. The nervous system picks up information through sensory and chemical receptors and, in turn, sends the appropriate stimulus back to your body's cells. The nervous system that sends messages to the brain to make your heart contract and beat also signals your brain to tell it your heart is broken and not to trust.

The enteric nervous system is a mesh-like system that lines your gut. Our common language and expressions, such as "trust your gut" or "I knew it in my gut," has long held the understanding that our gut holds knowledge. These are the feelings we should trust and honor; they reveal our deep visceral understanding of the stomach and brain connection. This function is now a prominent area of research in Western biomedicine.

As scientists learn about spiritual truths, they are learning that the memory bank in our brain holds cellular memory and each of our nerve cells at their synapses *also* stores memory. For example, our uterine nerve cells have memory, and our liver's nerve cells also hold memory. Specific memories can temporarily paralyze us because our overtaxed, traumatized nervous system will not respond to messages sent to move or act. The body has

learned to shut down. This response is how trauma can live in the body. While we may not be going through the wounding in the present time, the stored memory enables us to believe that we are experiencing trauma in the here and now.

Plants for the Nervous System

Nervous system plants are as diverse and dynamic as the nervous system itself. Stress can manifest in many places in the body, so our plants reflect that specificity. They are plants that support the central nervous system, the brain, and the spinal cord. Some plants work to support the enteric nervous system found in the gut. Others help the peripheral nervous system found in our extremities. Based on what the body is experiencing, we can choose the plant support we need.

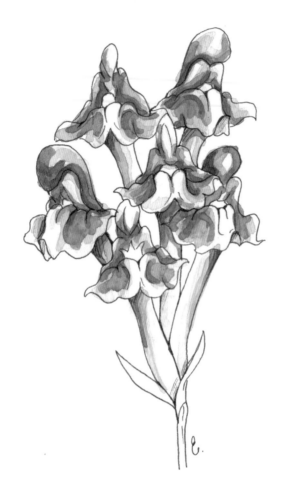

SKULLCAP

Skullcap is useful for central nervous system issues, such as stress and anxiety, and many diseases associated with stress in our bodies. One of my apprentices calls this the gateway herb. She says if you take skullcap, you will believe in herbal medicine.

A stern caregiver and parent, skullcap is a fierce protective force that grounds an overactive nervous system. It's medicine that is needed now because of its intensity, going straight to an issue like an arrow. It helps handle the immediacy of change.

Skullcap is cooling and great for hot conditions such as anxiety and panic attacks. Skullcap helps keep you centered and your central nervous system calm while everything around you might be spinning. It provides stillness in the middle of the storm so you can maintain perspective.

The energy of this herb is Saturn and Water, which makes perfect sense. Saturn is about building structures. Water has its structure in the form of ice. Skullcap is beneficial when we need to freeze everything around us. It helps us remain cool and get things done regardless of outer circumstances. Like water, it also teaches how discipline in fluidity can look. It feels like a cooling flow that encourages stillness even within the storm.

Common Name: Skullcap

Latin Name: *Scutellaria lateriflora*

Other Names: Maddog, Madweed, Helmet Flower

Taxonomy: Lamiaceae

Botanical Description: This perennial plant in the mint family has thin, ovate, lanceolate leaves and blue flowers.

Native Habitat: North America; grows in damp places, meadows, and roadside ditches

Wildcrafting and Cultivation: Sow by seed in damp conditions; requires full sun. Gather stems and all aerial parts when not flowering.

Parts Used: Aerial parts (above ground), not the flower

Planetary Influence/Correspondence: Saturn, Water

Energetic Quality: Bitter, cool

Pharmacological Constituents: Flavonoids; bitter iridoids; volatile oils; tannins

Ethnobotanical/Historical Use: Skullcap was used extensively by the Cherokee to stimulate menses and bring the afterbirth or placenta. It cured rabies in the 1970s, which is why it's called maddog and madweed.

Actions/Properties: Central nervous system tonic; antispasmodic; lowers blood pressure; sedative; analgesic; emmenagogue

Indications: Anxiety; stress; high blood pressure; epileptic seizures; insomnia; conditions aggravated by stress; withdrawal from substances and habits; stress headaches; neuralgia; fevers; fright; shock; pain; and PTSD. Use a tonic of skullcap for someone who is exhausted mentally.

It is particularly good for someone with an over-stimulated nervous system if they are nearing a nervous breakdown and experience heart racing, tense muscles, and panic attacks.

Contraindications: During pregnancy, use skullcap in small amounts only in formulation with other herbs to balance its energy. Use caution if taking any mental health medications because it works on the same system. Do not use a skullcap during the day or while driving. It has a highly sedative effect.

Methods of Preparation and Dosage

Infusion: Steep 1 tablespoon (3 g) in 8 ounces (235 ml) hot water for 20 to 25 minutes. Use as needed.

Tincture: Use 15 to 30 drops of tincture 3 times a day.

LEMON BALM

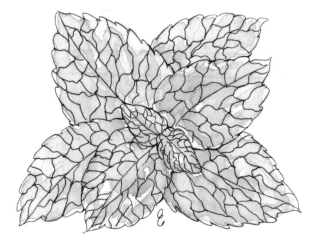

Lemon balm has always been a favorite of my daughter, Lauren. When she was little, we would brew lemon balm tea by the light of the Moon, leaving it outdoors overnight. We would drink it first thing in the morning while sharing our dreams. Lemon balm was Lauren's first herb. Throughout her life, we used lemon balm for any moments she felt stressed.

Lemon balm is a beautiful herb for children who are a part of the industrial complex that public education currently is. Lemon balm lemonade is a brilliant way to introduce it to children.

Lemon balm feels like a baptism of calm, sweet waters washing over you. This plant is guided by the Moon and Water, our primordial Mother, an herb of the river and ocean. Offer it to Oshun and Yemaya. Lemon balm is a gentle, cleansing herb because release can also be sweet like a bath from the Mother, an ocean bath, cleaning and renewing with gentleness.

Common Name: Lemon Balm

Latin Name: *Melissa officinalis*

Other Names: Bee Balm, Lemon Balsam, Sweet Melissa

Taxonomy: Lamiaceae

Botanical Description: Lemon balm features bright green, lemon-scented square stems with opposite leaves and small pale flowers that are white to cream in color.

The Art & Practice of SPIRITUAL HERBALISM

Native Habitat: Eastern Mediterranean; Europe; Central Asia; naturalized in the United States

Wildcrafting and Cultivation: Lemon balm grows like a weed. You should not wildcraft lemon balm from roadsides. Gather after or before flowering from clean and unsprayed areas at least 50 feet (15.2 m) away from the road. Sow by seed in January. Lemon balm likes to grow in full or partial sun.

Parts Used: Leaves and essential oils

Planetary Influence/Correspondence: Moon, Water

Energetic Quality: Pungent, sweet, cool

Pharmacological Constituents: Citrol; bitter principle; tannins; acids; flavonoids

Ethnobotanical/Historical Use: Lemon balm was revered as an elixir of life, and the physicians of old believed it chases away melancholy.

Actions/Properties: Diuretic; calming; emmenagogue; antidepressant; nervine; antimicrobial; antiviral; nutritive; thyroid balancer; tonic

Indications: Attention deficit disorder (ADD); upset stomach; stress; anxiety; tension; stress headaches; good for focus in children; calms and centers; good for fevers; postpartum blues; bipolar disorder; strong antiviral properties, specifically for herpes simplex

Contraindications: Do not use lemon balm during the late stages of glaucoma, as it can raise ocular pressure.

Methods of Preparation and Dosage

Standard Infusion: Steep 1 tablespoon (3 g) lemon balm in 1 cup (235 ml) water for 20 to 25 minutes. Drink freely up to 1 quart (1 L) per day of the standard infusion. My favorite preparation is as a Moon tea. Brew your tea as a standard infusion and set it out under the light of the full Moon. It is a delicious way to connect with the energy of this herb that is ruled by the Moon and Water.

Tincture: Use 15 to 30 drops of tincture 3 times a day.

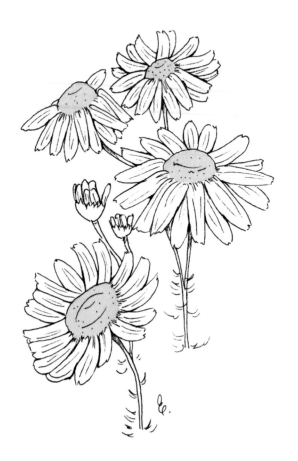

CHAMOMILE

Chamomile is brilliant for the stress we hold in our digestive system. This herb is for you when you are stressed and instantly nauseous or have cramps in the digestive system. Chamomile is an excellent herb premenstrually for headaches and pain that becomes difficult to bear.

I love the relationship it has with mothers and babies. Mom can drink chamomile and pass it to her baby through her breast milk. Chamomile is the quintessential baby herb and excellent for our childhood issues. We all go through our moments of wanting to be babied. Our inability to express, articulate, or obtain our needs can cause our actions to be that of a baby or a child. When those moments arrive, we can use chamomile. Use it in a bath when you feel prickly and fretful and when nothing can meet your needs.

Chamomile can ground you to prepare you for change. It calms your nervous system and offers space to hear and listen, giving you time to check in before taking that next step to move forward.

Common Name: Chamomile

Latin Name: *Matricaria recutita* (German Chamomile) and *Anthemis nobilis* (Roman Chamomile)

Other Names: Ground Apple, Wild Chamomile, Whig Plant, Manzanilla

Taxonomy: Asteraceae

Botanical Description: Chamomile features finely divided leaves and small daisy-like, sweet-scented white flowers that are yellow when dried. The German variety is annual, and the Roman variety is perennial.

Native Habitat: Europe; West Asia; India; naturalized everywhere

Wildcrafting and Cultivation: Chamomile is easy to grow by seed; sow in January. Harvest when flowers come up. It loves the sun, contributes to the health of the garden, and helps care for plants that grow nearby.

Parts Used: Flower, essential oil

Planetary Influence/Correspondence: Sun, Water

Energetic Quality: Spicy, aromatic, bitter, neutral

Pharmacological Constituents: Essential oils; coumarins; flavonoids; tannins; bitter principle; calcium; tryptophan (relaxes the parasympathetic nervous system)

Ethnobotanical/Historical Use: Chamomile was used as a strewing herb in the Middle Ages. (Strewing was when herbs were thrown on the floor, walked on to release the scent, and served as natural protection against disease.) Chamomile or manzanilla is used extensively in Mexico-American medicine.

Actions/Properties: Bitter; aromatic; sedative; relaxant; nervine; anodyne; antibacterial; anti-inflammatory; carminative; febrifuge; diaphoretic; stomatic; antihistamine; anticancer

Indications: Stress-related digestive issues; stomach pain; insomnia; stress; mild pain and inflammation; ulcers; gastritis; colic; mental and physical tension and spasms; canker sores; gum disease; pink eye; eye inflammation

Contraindications: No contraindications. However it does not support the first trimester of pregnancy. Be careful if taking antianxiety or other calming medications. More than 2 cups (475 ml) of the infusion can act as an emetic (make you throw up).

Methods of Preparation and Dosage

Infusion: Chamomile is best when prepared as a tea. (German chamomile is more often used for medicinal teas, while many garden varieties of chamomile are Roman chamomile.) Steep 1 tablespoon (3 g) in 1 cup (235 ml) boiling water for 20 to 25 minutes. The fresh infusion is best for calming nerves, and the dried infusion is better for digestive issues.

External Uses: Use chamomile as an eyewash for inflammation, or a face wash for acne. Use chamomile as a bath for babies who are irritable because of teething or earaches. It also promotes restful sleep. It is a good hair rinse for blonde highlights and dandruff.

ADDITIONAL PLANTS

Oatstraw *Avena sativa*

One of my favorite nervines, oatstraw is highly restorative to the nerves and nutrientdense. The plant is rich in B-complex vitamins and magnesium, required for the nervous system's healthy functioning. It nourishes and protects the myelin sheaths surrounding our nerves, ensuring the nervous system's smooth functioning. It is perfect for our culture at this time.

I especially recommend oatstraw when addressing burnout, grief, sudden shock, and trauma. It supports those involved in social-justice movements as it builds resistance and resilience to stress. It is also nourishing and restorative to individuals whose nerves feel dry and brittle from the effect of long-term stress. Oatstraw is helpful when you feel like you need support but don't have people or systems around you to provide it.

Contraindications: None

Tulsi (Holy Basil) *Ocimum sanctum*

Tulsi is an ancestral plant for me. When I was growing up in Guyana, tulsi was everywhere in my village. Grown as an offering to the Divine, tulsi is revered. It is used in prayer ceremonies to receive blessings from the Divine: from here, my reverence for this plant comes, and it is from this space I teach tulsi.

Often called the queen of herbs, tulsi is an adaptogen. An adaptogen is an herb that supports both the immune and the nervous systems. Adaptogens are often used as a tonic and can anticipate stressors in the body and protect against them.

Tulsi leaves and flowers are a digestive nervine, nourishing the nerves in the digestive tract. They are warming and soothing and support the breakdown of food and ridding the body of gas. Tulsi's use improves mood disorders, including anxiety and depression. I have used tulsi to gain clarity in thinking and enhance focus. Tulsi's scent is intoxicating, and just having it around can improve your mood and bring divine blessings.

Contraindications: Do not use if taking blood-thinning medications or have low blood sugar.

Passionflower *Passiflora incarnata*

My favorite thing to teach about this herb, commonly known as maypop, is that it is useful for list-making at night when your body needs rest. My herbal teachers taught me that passionflower eases the mind when thinking becomes repetitive as if on a loop.

This herb is mostly used as a sleep aid, as indicated for insomnia and anxiety. Passionflower might be too strong of a relaxant for some during the day. Others have found it to be helpful throughout the day when managing nervous tension and tension headaches. I have recommended this herb for the anxiety associated with withdrawal from substances like alcohol and cigarettes.

Contraindications: Not recommended if taking an anticoagulant.

Catnip *Nepeta cataria*

Catnip for humans?! I cannot tell you the number of times I have answered this question at Sacred Vibes Apothecary. Customers are very aware of the euphoric response of cats and not aware of the ways humans can consume catnip.

Catnip is a beautiful children's medicine. My son Zion has been referred to by many as the calmest person they know. Though there could be various reasons, I attribute his calmness to his love of catnip as a young toddler. He would drink a full cup of catnip infusion each night before bed and sometimes wake up asking for his tea. To this day, he leans on it for digestive relaxation and calming.

Catnip eases a child's fever, colic, sleeplessness, nervousness, hyperactivity, and irritability. It also works well in adults, as it aids indigestion and headaches caused by poor digestion. It is a favorite to add to an herbal smoking blend to strengthen the breath and voice.

Contraindications: Use with caution when taking sedative medications.

RECIPES

Beginning to Blend Herbs

The simplest way to begin to blend herbs as medicine is to take your time to get to know each herb's energy. Every herb should have a reason to be invited into your formulary. Understanding the energy, taste, and effects of the herb will help you determine what quantities to include, if at all. Some herbs are more potent than others and will naturally overpower the other herbs in a formula and therefore should be used in a much smaller quantity.

First begin by knowing why you are creating your formula. Is it for you? Is it for someone in your community or family? Why are you blending the herbs instead of using them as a single herb? What is the energy of the person you are making this medicine for? How old are they? Write it all down. When you have the answers to these questions, write out a recipe for your formula. How many parts of each herb should be used and why? Are you satisfied with how it feels? Have you used your intuition and knowledge of the plants you have selected to work with?

Once you feel good about your formula, begin with a minimal amount of herbs for each formula to avoid waste. Use a teaspoon as your measurement. Blend your mixture. Make a cup of tea and try it out. How does it look? How does it taste? Does any herb overpower the others? Would you want to drink this mixture daily? If you answer "yes," then make your formula in a larger quantity!

You can always adjust the mix based on your needs. Have confidence and trust yourself. Your mistakes are part of the learning process. Write every aspect of your process down. It's a great learning tool for an herbalist to review their early formulary. I love to go back and look at my formulary's early days that held so much simplicity and joy!

Inspired Sleep and Dreams Tea

This tea is used 20 minutes before bedtime to have inspire dreams. You can add honey to sweeten if you like.

1 tablespoon (3 g) dried lemon balm leaves

½ tablespoon dried mugwort leaves

1 tablespoon (3 g) dried chamomile flowers

1 tablespoon (3 g) dried damiana herb

1 tablespoon (3 g) dried lavender flowers

Honey (optional)

Yield: 4 cups (940 ml)

Mix the herbs together well. Store the blend in a mason jar. Prepare your tea each night before bed using 1 tablespoon (3 g) of the mixture to 1 cup (235 ml) boiling water. Cover and steep the infusion for 20 minutes. Strain and add honey if you would like. Drink 20 minutes before bed. Enjoy your dreams!

Inspired-Sleep Dream Pillow

I forever love using herbs under my pillow and my children's pillows to help with protection-enhancing dreams and protection from nightmares. Here is a simple blend of herbs that genuinely makes a difference. The rice is optional. Throughout African diasporic cultures, we have used rice as a protectant. Many of our ancestors were rice farmers and have built a strong relationship with rice. I include it here to honor that ancestral relationship and protection.

Use a few sprigs or tablespoons of the following herbs.

1 part chamomile flowers	1 part thyme leaves
1 part mugwort flowers	Rice (optional)
1 part rosemary leaves	**Yield:** 1 dream pillow

Combine the herbs in a muslin bag. Add the rice (if using). Tie the bag closed and place it under your pillow. Alternatively, you can bundle them and hang them near your bed or leave them on your nightstand as you sleep.

Inspired Sleep Dream Bath

An herbal bath releases the day's tension and prepares the body for rest and to enter the world of dreams. The herbs selected encourage relaxation and ease in falling asleep.

1 handful rosebuds	1 handful chamomile flowers
1 handful lavender flowers	**Yield:** 1 bath

Combine the herbs in a muslin bag and add them to your bathwater. Alternatively brew the herbs as a tea and add it to your bathwater.

Ancestral Practice: The Medicine of Dreams

The pineal gland is the part of the endocrine system that works closely with the nervous system. It is the link between Spirit and matter. This gland is responsible for much of our dreaming. Taking care of the pineal gland allows us to have lucid dreams and receive clear Spirit messages.

Your dreams, like your waking life, are another state of consciousness. They can show you what needs healing and what is coming. The indigenous believed that dreams don't represent things in our lives; instead, they are our lives in expanded perceptions. In our waking lives, we are present to physical manifestation. Our dream life can present a more subtle, albeit powerful, manifestation.

Our dreams can bring insight, clarity, and expansion to our waking life. They can offer us pieces of wisdom that contain insight into creating a path for our healing when we may see none. Healing work can happen in our dreams that we couldn't do in our daily lives, such as healing intergenerational trauma.

We can open up to new possibilities, ideas, visions, options, and outcomes through our dreams. We can consult our teachers, guides, and ancestors in our dreams to receive wisdom, assist with decisions, remember information, receive medicine, and heal our relationships.

Dreams can be used for problemsolving and holding visions within the collective, as the community also informs our dreams. They can inspire creativity and survival for our communities. Many indigenous cultures, including Native Americans, Africans, the people of ancient Kemet, Greece, China, and Rome, used dream interpretation for wellness, healing, and prevention of disasters in their communities.

A point to note is that nighttime is not the only time we dream, and we don't always have to go to sleep to dream. Daydreams and meditative dreams also hold tremendous insight and medicine for our healing.

Dreamtime

Prepare your space.

To encourage inspiration from Spirit, clear your body and mind before bed by taking a shower or bath. Cleanse your sleeping space by smudging with local plants. Garden sage and mugwort are excellent to clear and offer protection for your dream journey.

Set your intention.

Set your intention for a peaceful, protected sleep. You can utilize a dream tea (page 165) or a dream smoke (page 49). These medicines enhance the dreamworld's reality through lucid dreaming and help you remember your dreams.

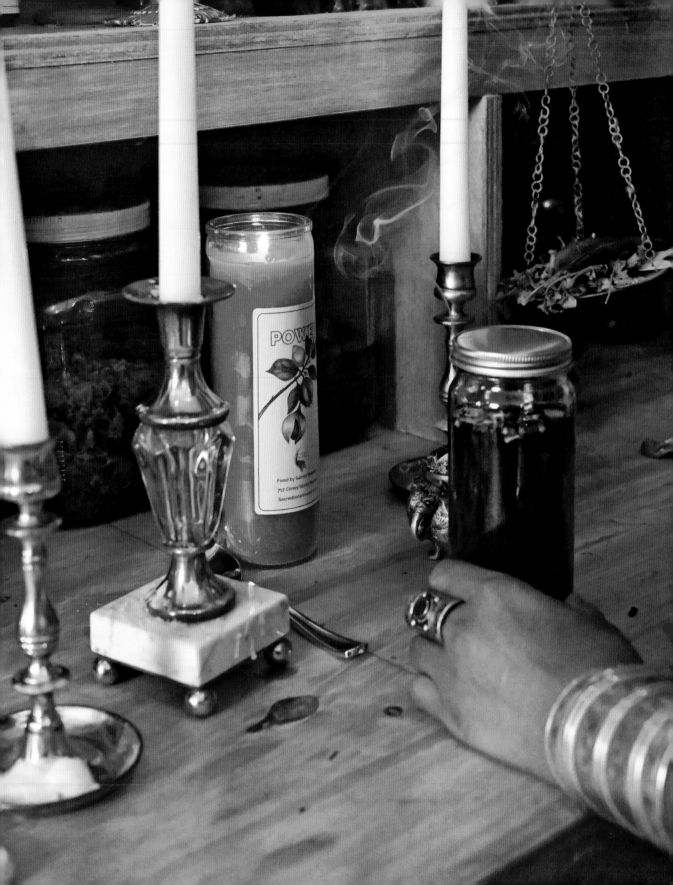

Call on your ancestors, guides, and angels.

Call on your ancestors and guides to be present, thanking them for the care they have shown you and asking them to watch over your dream space. You can sleep with a crystal such as black tourmaline or smoky quartz or plant medicine ally/allies, such as the dream pillow (page 166), to feel more protected.

Express gratitude.

With each breath, state positive affirmations and give thanks for the day that is ending. If there are specific questions, ask them now in your mind. And leave them there for the answers to come in your dreams.

Journal your dreams.

Upon waking, write down your dreams, share them with a trusted partner, or record them. Sharing imprints them into our waking consciousness. Dreamwork is like any other practice: You must be patient as it gets better with time. Don't be discouraged should you not remember your dreams at first.

Review your journal.

After a week, revisit your journal and notice common themes, people, places, colors, objects, and animals. Notice your age, gender, appearance, and feelings in your dreams. Notice how your waking reality informs your dreamtime.

Ask yourself questions.

As you review and reflect on your journal, your dreams bring you knowledge and innovative ideas? Were they a release for built-up emotions? Did your dreams bring messages from your ancestors, guides, or Spirit?

Remember that dreams are alive and, each time we visit them, we can learn something new.

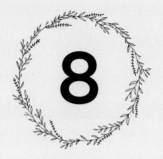

Protection!
IMMUNE HEALTH

———

The body is wise, and at its wisest and most magical is our immune system. I believe the extent of this system's work is still a mystery waiting for us to discover. Our immune system is our body's defense system against invaders—spiritual, emotional, and physical.

In Chinese medicine a large part of the immune system is our wei chi, the protective layer and energy force that guards our bodies. When your wei chi is healthy and nourished, you are impenetrable to viruses, pathogens, and other outside invaders, whether physical or spiritual.

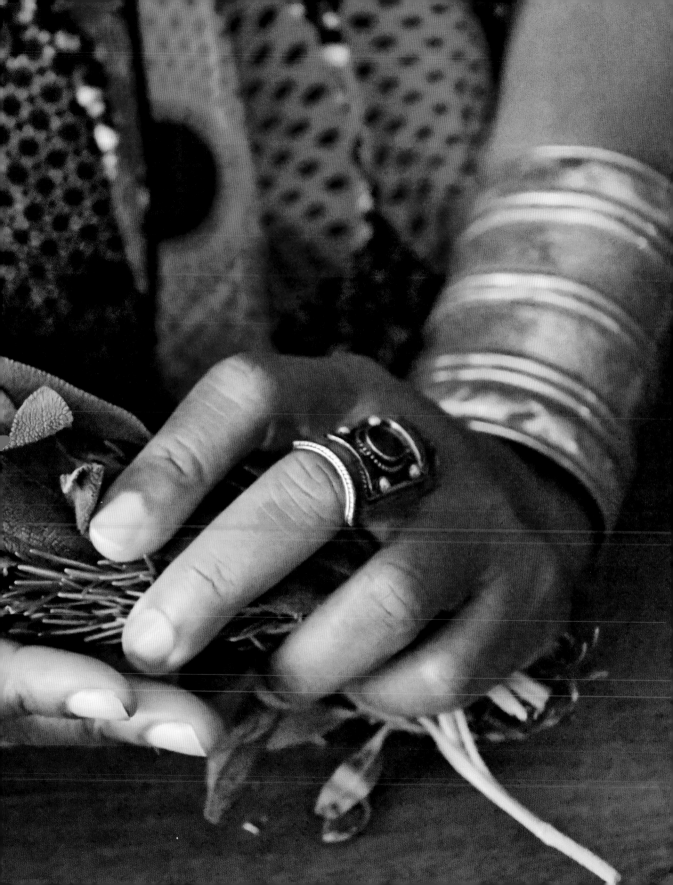

Our lifestyle and everyday stress diminish our wei chi. This absence, along with a lack of community support, forgiveness, and spiritual practice, creates an inability to assert and defend ourselves. Shoring up our wei chi is our daily work. I call this work protection work, and it is ongoing. It is preventative medicine and practices that we employ, not waiting until the immune system is compromised before we try to fix it.

Over my years as an herbalist, my apprentices will testify to my lengthy admonishment around protection work. Our days should start and end with calling in protection. I have marveled at how we choose our breakfast, choose our adornment for the day, and run out the door without our most crucial shield—protection! Protection is defined as a shield or barrier that protects you from suffering harm or injury.

Protection work is practicing prevention and strengthening our shield. Simply put, that shield is Spirit, divine forces, angelic guides, our ancestors, and our human body. When our relationship to these protective forces is lacking, we create external sources of security, a pseudoform of protection, and an expansion of colonized thinking called "boundaries" in the West.

Real protection is always spiritual and entirely different from boundaries. It is innate, the shield that exists around us that we walk through life, and it is strengthened by our spiritual connection and our body's health.

The immune system is coguided by the planets Mars and Neptune. The energy of Neptune unites humanity in oneness and love. It is about extending compassion and dissolving boundaries. When boundaries dissolve, we open to everything, including viruses and emotional and spiritual attacks. We are moving toward a more united global community, with the removal of borders and boundaries, toward a dissolution of independence and upliftment of interdependence.

As these Neptunian developments happen, we will witness the rise of new viruses that demand that the immune system evolves along with us into a more compassionate understanding of what protection can look like without borders and boundaries.

The Western concept of boundaries seeds itself on the creation of more. The more we have, the more we need, and the more we think that we are protected. It is a damaging and false concept that the more boundaries we institute, the more protected we are. Boundaries, as taught, are rooted in a lack of community. Much of our healing professionals' training and education in the West centers around boundary creation.

As healers, we have created boundaries that prevent us from acting from a heart-centered place. Many times our walls keep us from opening up and connecting heart to heart. As healers, we have to be accessible. Relationship building is the foundation for healing. People recognize truth and know when we are withholding, and this damages the opportunity to have a real connection, empathy, compassion, and true healing.

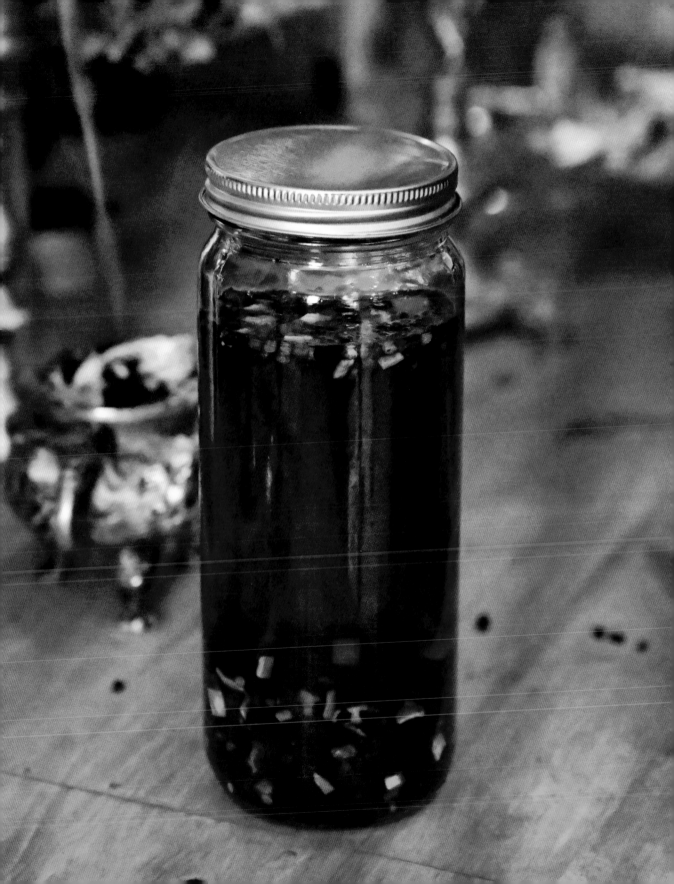

The Spirit of Protection

Energy of Fire: Mars, or the energy of orisha Oggun, is that of a warrior. It is a natural protective energy that speaks to us as the need to defend and protect ourselves. Oggun manifests as the courage we have in our convictions and the ability to live our purposes out loud. Our immune system relies on us being fierce, purposeful, outspoken, and bold.

If you regularly come down with colds, flu, and other viral infections, assess your ability to assert yourself. Are you able in your life to ask for what you deserve, at work, at home, with your partners, or with your parents? Are you able to stand in your power?

Unbalanced Martial energy often shows up in the way our immune system responds. Individuals identified as Aries Sun, rising, or Moon will do well to consider how they are balancing this dynamic energy. As Oggun, Mars is pure fire, and to remain balanced, we have to learn how to be keepers of our fire. Where is it burning too hot or where has it dimmed or completely snuffed out?

Energy of Water: The energy of Neptune or orisha Olokun is that of the visionary, the mystic, and the one who has achieved spiritual sight. This energy is precisely the motivation we need to move us forward in creating the world as we dream it, a relational and united world. The dreamworld is part of our protection. The pituitary gland, the master gland of our endocrine system, is responsible for our spiritual sight, regulating our dreaming, and playing a significant role in our immune system. Indigenous culture knew that our dreams held signals and warnings from the ancestors that would shield us in our daily lives.

Olokun lives at the base of the ocean, our subconscious, and holds many mysteries—things we have not yet tapped into in our consciousness. The ocean, our emotions, is vast and wide, and some things that lie at the base of our emotions have not yet consciously surfaced and ultimately determine our reactions. Being tapped into this mystery means awareness and self-knowing, self-forgiveness, releasing being the victim, and letting go of feelings of shame and blame.

Practicing forgiveness strengthens the immune system. Our inability to forgive can provide the basis for an autoimmune disorder. Unable to let go of old hurts can affect how we heal. Accepting our part in any situation requires courage and honesty. Our ability to see our role releases us from victimhood or martyrdom.

Neptune's energy diffuses individuality into oneness, which makes us feel connected to everyone and everything. This energy warps in ways that have us not knowing where we end and where another begins—creating the toxic dynamic of being a savior, needing a savior, or being a martyr. Healing means realizing that you are your savior and the redeemer you've been waiting on. Our ability to have autonomy and ownership over our lives is a protective shield.

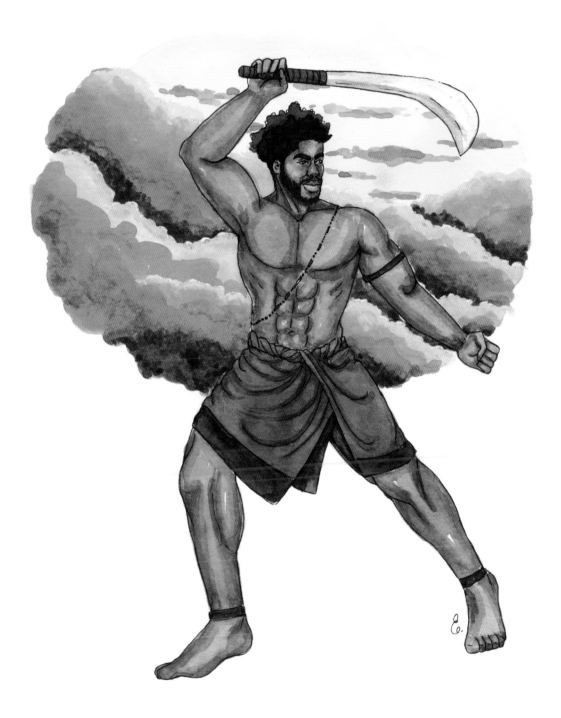

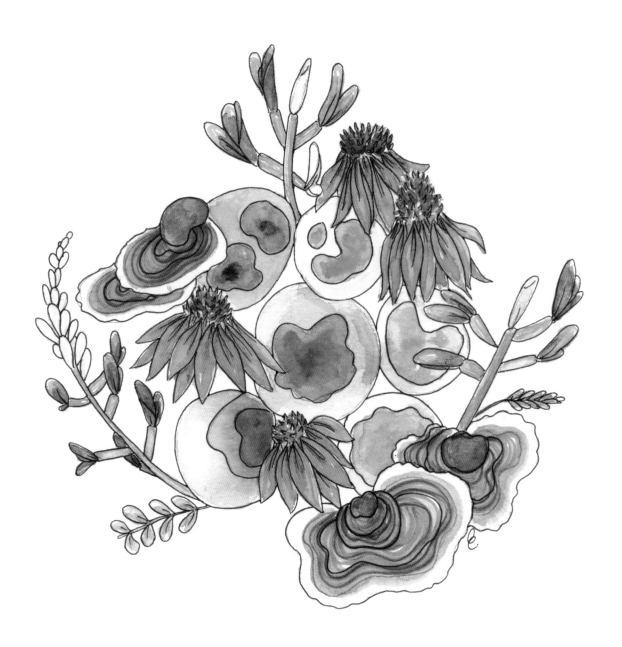

The Art & Practice of SPIRITUAL HERBALISM

Blame and shame are negative emotions that cause illness. In indigenous African cultures, shame is like death. No one is perfect. Quit aiming for perfection and being self-critical. To be perfect doesn't mean to be healed. To be whole means to be healed. Wholeness and perfection are two different things. Look at the standards you have for yourself that are unreachable and how you can be hard on yourself. When this happens, you create a breakdown in your immune response.

Though this energy seems inconsistent with the energy of Oggun, which asks us to stand in the power of our individuality, the energy of Olokun asks us to merge. Individuality is not independence; independence is contrary to our indigenous minds. Indigeneity encourages interdependence as a means of survival. Individuals who stand in their purpose come together to create a communal purpose, which is protective to the community. Olokun and Oggun's energy complement the individual's spiritual growth, where knowledge of self includes knowing ways to protect while yet remaining open.

Immune System

Our complex immune system includes the thymus gland, the spleen, the body's lymphatic system, and bone marrow. Our daily activities support the immune system's health, including getting adequate rest, eating a clean diet, drinking enough water, breathing clean air, reducing stress, and moving our bodies.

Teaching this was much needed during the COVID-19 pandemic because, at that time, people panicked and sought whatever they felt could improve their immune system overnight. As herbalists and healers, we had to reiterate that the immune system's complex design connects to the body as a whole and that our care for all aspects of our bodies creates a healthy immune system. Gut health, dental health, the liver's health, the kidneys, and the colon are all part of a robust immune system.

Stress depresses the immune system. Many people come into Sacred Vibes Apothecary after being ill and connect between their illness and their recent stress. We can overtire ourselves due to our exhausting schedules. Even with good intentions, we can exhaust our bodies. When we are stressed, our protective shield is weak and wide open to invaders.

Over the years in my practice I have seen that aggressive autoimmune conditions often respond to the boundaries we have created. Capitalism breeds aggression and aggressive attitudes, which often leads to overactive immune system responses. Hypervigilance treats our healthy organs as a problem, and our immune system overworks to protect us. Allergies are an expression of such a response. Healing requires vulnerability, moving beyond our positions of safety into courageous expressions and action.

The opposite of that is someone who has an underactive immune response. Diseases such as multiple sclerosis (MS) and chronic fatigue syndrome link to an underactive immune response. They manifest as depression, lack of focus, and low energy. This is an absence of passion, energy, will, purpose, and desire—all things that Oggun represents, the fire and will to be strong in your individuality.

Whenever you are working with an underactive immune system, ask yourself what you are passionate about. What is it that you desire most to do, and what are the blockages in your way that repress your ability to assert yourself in this world? It is our job to figure out what our passions are and create our world.

Understand that anger is not a disease. Know that we can be passionate, angry, and lustful, emotions that we have taught are unbecoming and learn to stifle inside. Healing means finding ways to be comfortable with the range of our feelings and to express them. Accept that anger is a part of our human response and what makes us human. And when ignored, it then has control over us.

Plants for the Immune System

Plants that support the immune system protect and shield our vital energy force that surrounds the body while opening us up to receive more light. The immune system requires light, the light of Spirit. We have all seen the effects of sunlight and vitamin D on the immune system. These plants support us by leaning into spiritual connection, building our chi, and offering fierce protection.

Both reishi and astragalus are adaptogens and immune modulators when used over time. Adaptogens are essential for healing the immune systems, as they work to anticipate stressors that could be facing the body while strengthening the immune system. No Western medicine does this. Yes, plants are magical.

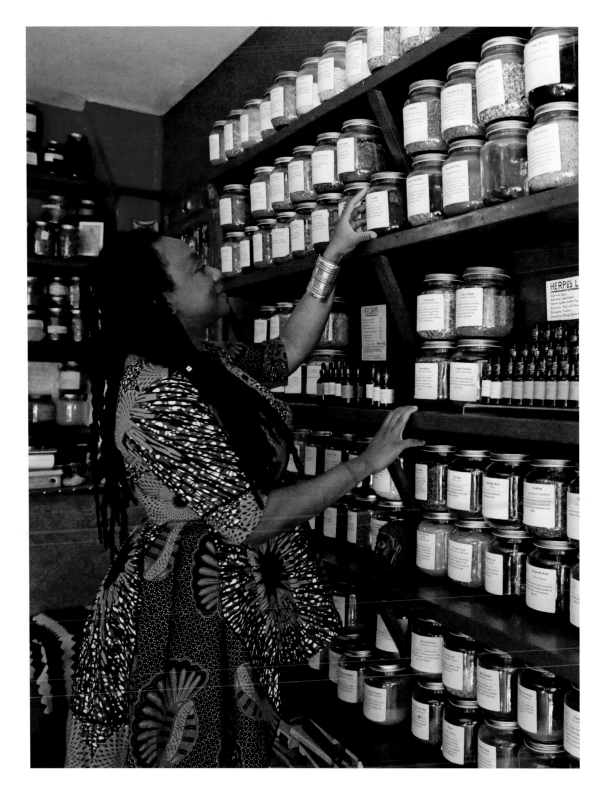

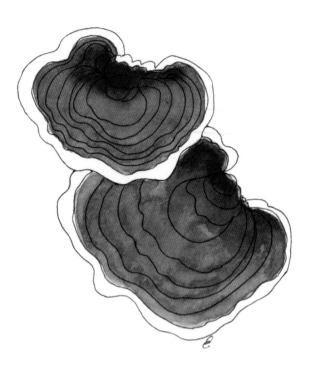

REISHI

One of reishi's common names is the red pill mushroom. Yes, like in the movie The Matrix where the blue pill is the return to "normalcy" where nothing changes, and the red pill, well, that opens your eyes and changes your life forever. The choice is ours. We can choose to live our lives without the truth, or we can choose to see the reality of our lives and our world. There is no going back after this clarity of sight, and this is the power of reishi, the bringer of light.

Traditionally used by shamans, reishi heightens mental perception. Its genus name, *Ganoderma*, means "bright shining," and its species name, *lucidum,* means "light." Lucidum is associated with Lucifer in the Bible, the angel of light with much access to knowledge. Lucidum/light or la luz is related to the Moon's light and the wisdom it holds.

Reishi—called the elixir of life and more treasured than gold—is one of my favorite adaptogens. Because of the immune system's intelligence, it feels equally important to match that intelligence with mushrooms' magic, in this case, reishi. In traditional Chinese medicine, reishi has been used to balance the mind and heal spiritual illnesses that we would call mental illnesses. Reishi supports clarity and creates insight, self-awareness, and spiritual potency.

Common Name: Reishi

Latin Name: *Ganoderma lucidum*

Other Names: Red Pill Mushroom, Ling Zhi, Soul Mushroom, Nourish Spirit Mushroom

Taxonomy: Ganodermataceae

The Art & Practice of SPIRITUAL HERBALISM

Botanical Description: Reishi is an annual fungus with a yellow to dark red fan-shaped body. The red mushrooms are best for medicine.

Native Habitat: China; abundant in Upstate New York on living and dead oak trees

Wildcrafting and Cultivation: You can gather reishi in the wild, but don't take it all, or the strongest ones, and make sure you can make a positive identification. Many mushrooms are poisonous. Reishi is often found growing on dead oaks. You can inoculate logs with reishi spores.

Parts Used: Mushroom

Planetary Influence/Correspondence: Uranus, Jupiter, Earth

Energetic Quality: Bland, sweet, bitter, neutral to warm

Pharmacological Constituents: Polysaccharides; phytosterols; terpenes; triterpenes; proteins; adenosine

Ethnobotanical/Historical Use: In China, reishi has been considered an elixir of life. Reishi has been introduced to Western herbalism from traditional Chinese medicine in the last thirty years.

Actions/Properties: Adrenal restorative; metabolic; antiaging; oxygenator; immune modulator; antitumor; anticarcinogenic; antiviral; antiallergic; hepatoprotective; nervine; adaptogen; antioxidant; regulates cholesterol; inhibits blood platelet malfunction; helps with radiation; tonic to the parasympathetic nervous system; tonic to the adrenal cortex of the kidneys

Indications: Immune deficiency; allergies; chemotherapy; chemo recovery; cardiac stress; insomnia; heart palpitations; ADD and ADHD; mental health issues; mushroom poisoning; chronic degenerative disease

Contraindications: Do not use in those with sensitivity to mold.

Methods of Preparation and Dosage

Reishi yields its properties best through a water decoction.

Decoction: Use 1 ounce (28 g) reishi to 9 cups (2.1 L) water. Bring to a boil and then reduce the heat to let simmer for 2 to 3 hours as it reduces to one-third of its volume or 3 cups (705 ml). The mushrooms can be reused at least one other time. Store it in the freezer between uses.

Reishi is introduced slowly to the body. Drink ⅓ cup (80 ml) decoction 2 to 3 times per day on an empty stomach, 20 to 30 minutes before eating. As your body builds up its tolerance to the medicine, you can increase it to ½ cup (120 ml), then 1 cup (235 ml), 2 to 3 times a day.

Tincture: Take 15 to 30 drops of tincture 3 times per day.

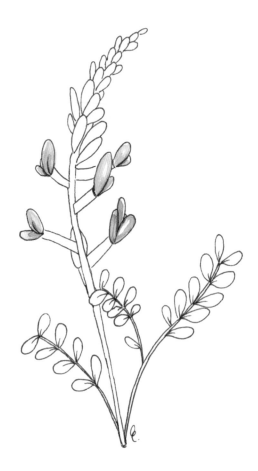

ASTRAGALUS

Another of my favorite adaptogens is astragalus, an herb we reach for several times a day at Sacred Vibes Apothecary. Astragalus strengthens and repairs the body's wei chi, the protective force that surrounds the body. It is a profoundly nourishing herb, an adaptogen that can shield us in times when we need extra protection.

Astragalus is restorative and is excellent for healers who give without receiving or pouring back into their self-nourishment. It reminds us that when we feel protected and shielded, we need fewer boundaries. This herb helps protect from emotional depletion, giving too much, and leaking vital energy. Its medicine is magical for those within systems that serve, such as nurses, educators, and students. I love to recommend it to those involved in evolution/revolution work, including movement building and accountability uprisings.

It is everyday preventative medicine for our bodies and is especially great for chronic illnesses that wear us down over time. Astragalus is food and does not interfere with prescription drugs. Its constituents are that of many nutritious root vegetables and is used by the body in the same way.

Many of my students have experimented with ways to incorporate this root into their diet. Some of the favorites I have heard are astragalus included in daily oatmeal blends, porridges, cooking broths, and soups. Use powdered astragalus root in muffins or cookies and prepare grains in an astragalus decoction.

Astragalus is a tonic herb and can be taken throughout the winter months to strengthen the immune system.

The Art & Practice of SPIRITUAL HERBALISM

Common Name: Astragalus

Latin Name: *Astragalus membranaceus*

Other Names: Life Energy Builder, Huang Qi, Milk Vetch

Taxonomy: Fabaceae

Botanical Description: This perennial herb has long, pale yellow roots, divided leaves, pale yellow flowers, and kidney-shaped seeds.

Native Habitat: North Central China; Inner Mongolia

Wildcrafting and Cultivation: Gather the roots in autumn, slice them lengthwise, and chop them up. Can be grown on the East Coast; collect it in early fall in well-drained/sandy alkaline soil.

Parts Used: Roots

Planetary Influence/Correspondence: Jupiter, Mars, Air

Energetic Quality: Sweet, warm, dry

Pharmacological Constituents: Polysaccharide; flavonoids; saponins; alkaloids

Ethnobotanical/Historical Use: Traditional Chinese medicine used astragalus in the fall for people who work outside during the winter because it braces the kidneys, improves function of the bone marrow, and builds immunity.

Actions/Properties: Immune builder; adrenal tonic; blood tonic; cardiac tonic; adaptogen; antibacterial; antihydratic; antihypertensive; anti-inflammatory; antiviral; diuretic; immune stimulant; strengthens the body's protective chi

Indications: Kidney yang deficiencies; chronic issues; compromised immune system; fibromyalgia; multiple sclerosis (MS); low energy; frequent colds; diabetes; exhaustion; hypertension; organ prolapse; poor sperm motility; AIDS; HIV; hepatitis; tumor growth; restores immune function after steroid use

Contraindications: Not to be used for acute symptoms when infection is present; it can drive the infection deeper. Recommended for chronic illness and long-term use.

Methods of Preparation and Dosage

Decoction: Simmer 1 tablespoon (3 g) astragalus in 2 cups (475 ml) water for 25 minutes. Drink 1 cup (235 ml) of tea 3 times a day.

Tincture: Use 1 dropper or 30 drops of tincture 3 times a day.

Powered Root: Use 1 teaspoon 3 times a day as an everyday preventative. The root can be added to smoothies, porridge, oatmeal, etc.

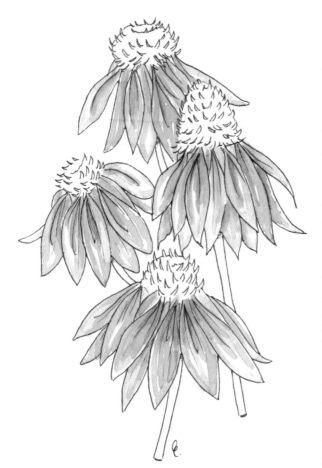

ECHINACEA

Echinacea is an endangered plant and potent medicine. At the turn of the twentieth century, echinacea was the most used herbal remedy, and 100 years later, it remains. There is tremendous misuse of this most valuable plant medicine. People believe that they should take echinacea as an ongoing tonic, which is countereffective to the immune system's functioning. It stimulates the immune system to react to a pathogen entering the body. Echinacea is strong medicine for acute conditions, not chronic ones. Take echinacea at the first signs of illness from viral infections such as colds and flu. Symptoms rarely persist after a ten-day round of echinacea; use other herbs to clear any persistent symptoms.

Echinacea, used by the native people of this land for venomous snakes, offers enhanced spiritual protection. Its removal of energy is exact and effective as though extracting the venom of a snake. What needs to be extracted and exorcised from your life? What is the spirit/energy you are walking with that is not your own and needs removal? We move through this world with much attached to us that is not of our origin. Echinacea removes these unwanted energies.

In our apprenticeship program, we liken echinacea to spiritual surgery where the incision is precise, cutting away at what is poisoned and infected, leaving us whole.

Common Name: Echinacea

Latin Name: *Echinacea purpurea* and *Echinacea angustifolia*

Other Names: Snakeroot, Black Samson, Purple Coneflower

Taxonomy: Asteraceae

The Art & Practice of SPIRITUAL HERBALISM

Botanical Description: Echinacea is a perennial with sturdy, bristly haired stems, long black roots, and single flowers.

Native Habitat: Northeast United States and Midwest prairies; originally grown from Kansas to Montana and south to Oklahoma, and now grown coast to coast

Wildcrafting and Cultivation: Echinacea is overharvested. Do not gather in the wild as it is easily cultivated.

Parts Used: Roots and flowers (gentle but similar action)

Planetary Influence/Correspondence: Mars, Fire

Energetic Quality: Bitter, pungent, cool, dry

Pharmacological Constituents: Alkaloids; polysaccharides; essential oils

Ethnobotanical/Historical Use: Native communities in the U.S. plains used echinacea for snakebite, bug bites, and in sweat lodges to cool and create a numbing effect. Used by the Kiowa and Cheyenne people for coughs and sore throats. Used by the Pawnee for headaches. Many native communities, including the Sioux, used echinacea as an analgesic.

Actions/Properties: Alterative; antibiotic; antiseptic; antiviral; anodyne; anticatarrhal; antifungal; antitumor; carminative; diaphoretic; stimulant; immune stimulant; vulnerary; anti-inflammatory; lymphatic; inhibits viral replication

Indications: Microbial infection (e.g., strep throat; staph infection; tooth; gum and mouth infections); blood poisoning; urinary tract infection; septic fever; mastitis; sinusitis; bronchitis; chronic and acute sore throat; surgical and accidental wounds; stimulates formation of leukocytes; boils; acne; insect bites; colds; flu; viruses; lymph congestion and sluggishness; candida; Lyme disease; herpes, during periods of high stress for preventing and shortening outbreak; exhausted and depressed immune system; swollen veins in legs and arms

Contraindications: Overactive immune system; autoimmune issues; anyone on immunosuppressant drugs (can wear out immune system because it is so stimulating); leukemia; vertigo; dizziness; cold and dry systems

Methods of Preparation and Dosage

Echinacea is medicine for acute symptoms and should be used for 7 to 10 days.

Decoction: Use 1 tablespoon (3 g) to 2 cups (475 ml) water. Bring water to a boil and simmer for 20 to 25 minutes. Drink ½ cup (120 ml) of tea 2 times a day. Root can be reboiled.

Tincture: Use 10 to 60 drops of tincture 3 times a day. Take 5 to 10 drops every 1 to 2 hours for acute symptoms, lessening the dosage as you get better, for a total of 7 to 10 days.

Topically: Echinacea leaves and flowers can be used in poultices, salves, compresses, and washes. Can be used to speed tissue repair and bites.

Mouthwash: The whole plant—roots, leaves, and flowers—can be used for sore gums and gingivitis; prepare a strong tea and rinse with it.

ADDITIONAL PLANTS

Elder *Sambucus nigra*

If I asked most people to name an herb they have used over the last year to build their immune system, I am confident I would hear elder as an answer. Elderberries provide a sweet and gentle medicine for the immune system. While the taste of this medicine is mild, its medicinal components are vital. Elderberries are a potent antiviral that begins their protective work by shielding the virus from even entering the body.

Elder is accessible. Elder trees grow in many of our communities, and the berries can be used as medicine when dried. Elder spiritually is true to its name, offering the protection of a familiar elder. Many compare its energy to a protective guardian or grandfather, shielding us from storms and connecting us to the land of the Faeries. The tree's wood makes magical wands that invoke protection upon their users.

This herb is a favorite of mine to use with my younger customers. I find that children respond well to the energy of elderberry. It is delicious and works its magic overnight in clearing a cold or the flu virus. It is my son Shiloh's favorite medicine. He would refer to his morning doses of elderberry syrup as his "good, good" medicine and refused to leave home in the winter months without it. Unlike astragalus or echinacea, use elderberries as a tonic preventative and as a treatment for cold and flu.

Though we primarily use this plant's berries, use the flower to drive out cold and flu symptoms by their diaphoretic nature.

Contraindications: Cook or dry elderberries before use. Fresh berries are a laxative. Do not use bark or root. Know the species and make a positive identification; there are many poisonous berries.

Fo-ti Root (He Shou Wu)
Polygonum multiflorum

Fo-ti root is a supreme nourisher and restores life and vitality to the body. This plant has a long history of use in Chinese medicine to build longevity. One of its common names is Black-Haired Mr. Woo because it is said to keep the hair black. I recommend fo-ti root for symptoms of profound depletion and burnout. Fo-ti addresses symptoms such as a disinterest in life, insomnia, depression, lack of libido and sexual disinterest, lower back pains, and blood deficiencies. All these symptoms are indicative of a depleted kidney yin chi. Fo-ti is restorative to the liver and kidneys, which restores overall strength to the immune system.

Spiritually fo-ti restores our energy force. It connects us to our most vital selves so we may release fear and live potently. It brings us back to the feelings of youth and freedom, a sense of our true essential self, without the layers that we have constructed for protection.

Fo-ti is an adaptogen and an immune system enhancer. It is a lymphatic decongestant that encourages health in the body's lymph glands, a vital part of the immune system. I use this medicine to heal ancestral trauma or the impacts of parental chi, where our body's protective shield might have been damaged even before our conception because of our parents and lineage's health and wholeness.

Contraindications: Liver and kidney disease; diarrhea and loose stools; pregnancy and breast/chest feeding and with young children; prescription medications; stomach pains; or over extended periods

Spilanthes *Spilanthes acmella*

My love of spilanthes has grown over the years. It is an easy plant to grow and very useful for viral infections. It is a brilliant replacement for its endangered cousin, echinacea. This plant's tingling effect when chewed demonstrates its work as a potent antiviral.

This medicine is native to Africa and has a history of being used by the Zulus. When I think of this plant's energy, it is precisely that of a warrior and a fierce protector. It teaches tenacity and resilience: each place that the nodes on the plant's stem touch it forms a root, reminding us to root wherever we are. This resilience is especially needed when experiencing new lands in the face of forced migration, as it provides a protective shield when making our way to our new home.

Its Mars/Fire, Oggun energy supports us, centering us in asking for our needs while protecting us from energetic spiritual attacks.

Spilanthes is an immune stimulator, antibiotic, antifungal, and antiseptic all in one plant! It remains one of my favorite medicines to use when traveling. It is especially great for killing gnat larvae that spread malaria, dengue/yellow fever, and elephantiasis. I often squeeze a few drops of the tincture into whatever water I am drinking, where access to clean water might not be easy. It's the plant I reach for when a toothache feels like it is coming on. Spilanthes is often called the toothache plant because of its action in numbing gums. It is an antibiotic and eases any infection at the site of the tooth or gum.

Contraindications: Immune-suppressing medicines; autoimmune disease; chemotherapy

The Process of Medicine Making

Making medicine is a sacred practice that centers on our creativity, reverence, and intuition. Please choose the time carefully: not while you are on the phone, watching television, upset, or not feeling your best. Set a time when you can be alone and hold the space sacred where you can be in meditation with the spirit of the plant that guides this healing and that to come. I teach my apprentices that medicine making is healing, just as taking medicine is healing. A large part of the medicine is you, and you're the alchemist practicing alchemy, a magical and transformative process.

Medicine making on the Moon or menstrual cycle can offer an excellent opportunity for dynamic connection with Spirit. You become a channel to universal energies. When feeling held and safe and protected, it can be a magical time to commune with your intuitive powers and create medicine for you and your community.

In a connected and embodied state, we put our energy into the preparation, offering a piece of ourselves with our medicines. If we feel most connected to our anger flowing through us, we can use that energy to make resistance medicine.

That remedy can feel like a homeopathic remedy where "like treats like" encourages understanding, motivation, and acceptance of the energies of anger. It can feel like it knows itself and finds the hidden corners of our psyche.

Fully enlist your creativity and use all the tools, gems, color therapy, Moon cycles, and magical methods that speak to you. All of my students can make echinacea tinctures using the same process, and each of their medicines tastes differently.

It is essential to keep a medicine log, where you can list the ingredients, methods of preparation, date and batch number, Moon cycle, menstruum, parts used, and amounts. Share your medicine and write down the feedback you receive. It is an integral part of refining your medicine-making skills.

How to Make a Tincture

Tinctures are extractions of plant materials using a menstruum, such as alcohol, glycerin, or vinegar. Tinctures are accessible and support our busy lifestyles. They are the best medicine for acute conditions that require multiple doses in a short time frame. Tinctures are helpful when administering medicine to children, the elderly, and pets. When it might not be possible to ingest a cup of tea, a few tincture drops are ideal. They are perfect when traveling because of their size and accessibility, not needing to find a stove to heat water for tea making. Tinctures have a long shelf life of approximately two years, allowing us to prepare them in advance of when we might need them.

• Clean glass jar

• Plant material (dried or fresh)

• Menstruum, such as alcohol, glycerin, or vinegar

• Materials to label your jar

Fill the jar one-third of the way with dried plant material. If using fresh plant material, fill the jar. Pour the menstruum over the plant material, filling the jar to the top.

Label the jar with the plant, menstruum, and date. Preparing the label is a great place to write your intentions on the medicine as it tinctures.

Let it sit in a cool, dark place for 6 to 8 weeks. Shake 2 to 3 times a week or whenever you walk by or think about it! Say prayers or an affirmation repeating your intention over your medicine as you shake it.

After 6 to 8 weeks, strain with cheesecloth, squeezing out the plant material and retaining the liquid. Discard the plant material.

Rebottle the tinctured liquid into a clean glass amber or dark bottle and label.

Note: If using vinegar to make your tincture, use a plastic cap or cover it with plastic wrap before putting on a metal cap. The vinegar will corrode the metal, making it impossible to open once done tincturing.

The Art & Practice of SPIRITUAL HERBALISM

Garden Protection Bundle

Making herbal smudge bundles is one of my favorite projects during the summer season when fresh plants are readily available. I usually choose the plants I am working with based on their spiritual properties. If I am working with protection, I choose plants such as sage, thyme, oregano, yarrow, and rosemary. I recommend working with common garden plants that are accessible and local versus choosing endangered plants from other communities or, as in white sage or palo santo, furthers cultural appropriation.

A few clippings of sage, thyme, or rosemary

Twine, string, or yarn

Yield: 1 bundle

Lay your plants out on your workspace and arrange them as you would like to see them when bundled. Bundle them tightly in one hand as you use your other hand to wrap the twine around the plants, starting from the base. Wrap the twine around the bundle a few times and make a knot. Continue wrapping the twine upward on the bundle until you are a few inches from the top. Now wrap it downward, meeting the original knot you made at the bottom. Tie them securely together. There you have it, a protection bundle!

You can dry the bundle as it is, or wrap it in newspaper to dry to hold the bundle's form and assist even drying. I have used both ways, without a preference. The drying process takes about 1 week. Once dry, your bundle is now ready for use.

Use your smudge bundle by smudging yourself and your home before morning prayers, to clean your altar tools, and upon returning home to clear any energy that might have attached to you.

Protection Spray and Hand Sanitizer

Living in New York City requires a protection spray. This spray is a favorite way to quickly clear my energy and bring in protection while traveling around the city. In my daily bag, there is always a 2-ounce (60 ml) bottle of protection spray. I have used it to clear my energy after riding the subway, and to protect myself when entering an environment that feels challenging. Lately I have used it as a hand sanitizer given the need for increased protection during COVID-19 precautions.

The protection spray is an effective way to clear the room before and after consultations. This recipe is easy to prepare and takes less than an hour. I recommend making it with children, family, and community.

1 ounce (28 ml) distilled water

½ ounce (14 ml) vodka

½ ounce (14 ml) liquid aloe vera gel

A few drops of essential oil indicated for protection (rosemary, sage, lavender, etc.)

Yield: 2 ounces (56 ml)

In a clean glass 2-ounce (60 ml) spray bottle, combine the water, vodka, and aloe vera gel. Add a few drops of each of the essential oils you have chosen to work with, not exceeding 20 drops for every 2 ounces of liquid. Shake well, label, and spray when needed. This spray has an approximate 1-year shelf life.

Immunity Chai Tea

I have been making an immunity tea every year for the last twenty or more years of being an herbalist. It's an autumn ritual for my family and me to have this immunity tea on hand throughout the colder months. Our customers at Sacred Vibes Apothecary also love this blend, giving us rave reviews on how it helps them fight off cold and flu viruses and even benefits those with mold allergies. And it tastes delicious! Enjoy this blend as a daily tea.

2 tablespoons (18 g) elderberries	1 star anise
1 teaspoon astragalus root	2 or 3 cardamom pods
⅛ teaspoon black pepper	Coconut milk
⅛ teaspoon cloves	Honey, maple syrup, or agave
1 cinnamon stick	**Yield:** 4 cups (940 ml)

Crush the herbs in a mortar and pestle before placing them in a pot. Cover with 5 cups (1.2 L) water and bring to a boil. Simmer for 25 minutes. Strain off the plant materials using a fine-mesh sieve. Discard the plants and retain the tea. Add the coconut milk and honey to taste. Store prepared tea in the refrigerator. It has a shelf life of 1 to 2 days.

"Good, Good" Medicine—Elderberry Elixir

This recipe is so close to my heart and one of the first herbal medicines I mastered while still an herbalism student. I would make this medicine and give it to everyone for the holidays. Each year I would hear back from people, asking when they could get more. This syrup is another medicine I have in my home throughout winter. As I have said, my son, Shiloh, gets 1 tablespoon of it in the mornings before going to school. It's his shield as he navigates this world in a Black boy's body.

I teach this recipe to my Level II apprentices as we are beginning to experiment with formulary. I advise them to lean into their creative abilities and trust their intuition to add more or pull back any of the spices mentioned here. As with cooking, let it be your creation that is a treat for you to take each day.

1 ounce (28 ml) elderberries	Honey or maple syrup
2 tablespoons (12 g) orange peel	Brandy
2 cinnamon sticks	**Yield:** About 6¼ cups (1470 ml)
½ teaspoon cloves	

In a clean pot, simmer the elderberries, orange peel, cinnamon, and cloves in 5 cups (1.2 L) water for 25 minutes. Strain off the plant materials, measure the liquid and return it to the pot.

Measure one-quarter volume of the liquid in honey and sweeten the mixture. Add brandy, which should measure one-quarter of the volume of the decoction and honey.

Stir well and store in a clean glass jar. Take 2 to 3 tablespoons (30 to 45 ml) of the syrup each day to keep your shield strong all winter long.

Store syrup in the refrigerator. Discard in 45 days or if there is mold present.

Ancestral Practice: Protection Prayers

Our enslaved ancestors knew that protection came from beyond the physical; much if not all of their protection was spiritual protection. Indigenous African spiritual practices such as Voodoo, Myal, Kumina, Obeah, and Hoodoo center on the necessary task of protecting their practitioners. There is no way one would debate the power of spiritual protection on the individual, familial, and communal work that was the Haitian Revolution.

Some of our ancestors' magic had to be veiled by Christianity, as in Santeria, where ritual practices evolved alongside Christianity. Many enslaved people attended churches and continued to practice their ancestral traditions. With that, our ancestors employed a mix of resources to call in protection.

One such source is the connection that Black people have to prayer. They turned to the power of Scripture, particularly the Psalms, over generations to call in protection on our family members as they move outside in the world. Black grandmothers have marked their Bibles open to protection prayers while burning candles on their altars to invoke the safe return of their children and grandchildren. They have prayed and laid their blessed hands on us that we may be guarded and guided as we make our way in the world. In the Caribbean these Psalms said out loud are often accompanied by splashes of white rum. With reverence for this practice, I too invoke the protection of Psalm 91 upon my children and me when needed.

One of the simple ways I call in daily protection is through affirmations, said aloud in front of my ancestral altar before walking out the door in the morning. This ritual can be as simple as saying the affirmation and offering water or coffee. It can also include lighting a candle and sitting before your altar to share your thoughts and receive messages for the day. I conclude my time there with thanksgiving and any of these affirmations to call in protection. Choose one that feels right to you and repeat it throughout the day whenever you need safety.

Prayers for Protection

"I have nothing to fear. My ancestors and my guardians go before me, making my way."

"The shield within me and without me is strong and infinite and protects me from all harm."

"I am surrounded by infinite love, wisdom, and protection."

The Unity Prayer for Protection has also served me well. It is a follows:

"The Light of God surrounds you. The Love of God enfolds you. The Power of God protects you. The Presence of God watches over you. Wherever you are, God is, and All is Well."

GLOSSARY

Adaptogens: Herbs that improves the body's ability to adapt, helping it adapt around a problem. They help the body avoid reaching a point of collapse or overstress. The core of this action lies in helping the body cope with external pressures by supporting the adrenal glands and pituitary gland function.

Alterative: Herbs that will gradually restore the proper function of the body's health and vitality. They were at one time known as "blood cleansers."

Amphoteric: Herbs that are both stimulants and relaxants. Amphoteric herbs work in accordance with what the body needs at that time.

Analgesic, Anodyne: Herbs that reduce pain when applied externally or taken internally.

Anthelmintic: Herbs that destroy or expel worms from the digestive system.

Antibilious: Herbs that help the body remove excess bile.

Anticatarrhal: Herbs that help the body remove excess catarrhal buildup in the sinus area or in other parts of the body.

Antiemetic: Herbs that reduce nausea and prevent vomiting.

Anti-inflammatory: Herbs that help the body combat inflammation.

Antilithic: Herbs that prevent the formation of stones or gravel in the urinary system and assist in their removal.

Antimicrobial: Herbs that help the body destroy or resist pathogenic microorganisms.

Antineoplastic, Anticancer: Herbs that work to prevent the spread of cancerous cells.

Antirheumatic: Herbs that reduce and prevent pain and inflammation in the joints.

Antispasmodic: Herbs that help prevent or ease spasms or cramps.

Antitumor: Herbs that prevent or inhibit the growth of tumors.

Antitussive: Herbs that reduce coughing.

Aperients: Herbs that are very mild laxatives.

Aromatic: Herbs that have a strong, often pleasant scent and stimulate the digestive system. They are often used to add aroma and taste to other medicines.

Astringent: Herbs that contract tissue by precipitating proteins and can thus reduce secretions and discharges. They contain tannins.

Bitter: Herbs that taste bitter and act as stimulating tonics for the digestive system through a reflex via the taste buds.

Cardiac tonic: Herbs that affect the heart.

Carminative: Herbs that are rich in volatile oils and their action stimulates peristalsis of the digestive system and relaxes the stomach, supporting digestion and helping with gas in the digestive tract.

Cholagogue: Herbs that stimulate the release and secretion of bile from the gallbladder. They also have a laxative effect on the digestive system because bile is our internally produced, all-natural laxative.

Demulcent: Herbs that are rich in mucilage and soothe and protect irritated or inflamed internal tissue.

Diaphoretic: Herbs that aid the skin in eliminating toxins and promoting perspiration.

Diuretic: Herbs that increase the secretion and elimination of urine.

Emetic: Herbs that cause vomiting, usually when taken in high dosage.

Emmenagogue: Herbs that both stimulate and normalize menstrual flow.

Emollient: Herbs that are applied to the skin to soften, soothe, and protect it. They act externally in a manner similar to the way demulcents act internally.

Expectorant: Herbs that support the body in the removal of excess amounts of mucus from the respiratory system.

Febrifuge, Antipyretic: Herbs that help the body bring down fever.

Galactagogue: Herbs that help breast/chest feeding people increase the flow of milk.

Hemostatic: Herbs that stop blood flow.

Hepatic: Herbs that tone and strengthen the liver and increase the flow of bile.

Hypnotic: Herbs that induce sleep (not a hypnotic trance).

Laxative: Herbs that promote the evacuation of the bowels.

Nervine: Herbs that have a beneficial effect on the nervous system and tone and strengthen it. Some act as stimulants, some as relaxants.

Nutritive: Herbs that deeply nourish the body.

Oxytocic: Herbs that stimulate the contraction of the uterus and help in childbirth.

Pectoral: Herbs that have a strengthening and healing effect on the respiratory system.

Rubefacient: Herbs that, when applied to the skin, cause a gentle local irritation to stimulate the dilation of the capillaries, increasing circulation to the skin. Blood is drawn from deeper parts of the body into the skin and internal pain is relieved.

Sedative: Herbs that calm the nervous system and reduce stress and nervousness throughout the body.

Sialagogue: Herbs that stimulate the secretion of saliva from the salivary glands.

Soporific: Herbs that induce sleep.

Stimulant: Herbs that quicken and enliven the physiological functions of the body.

Stomatic: Herbs that aid the stomach.

Styptic: Herbs that reduce or stop bleeding by their astringency.

Tonic: Herbs that strengthen and enliven either specific organs or the whole body.

Vulnerary: Herbs that, when used externally, help heal wounds and cuts.

RESOURCES

While there are many online sources for purchasing organic herbs, my focus is not on recommending wholesalers.

Community apothecaries. Owned by people who live in our communities, community apothecaries are worthy of our support. The work that we do in our apothecaries is sacred. The herbalist makes recommendations on the plants to support. You are listened to, honored, and partnered with you to address your healing. Get advice on dosage, contraindications, and preparations. The space of the apothecary builds, shapes, and heals communities alongside individuals.

Local farmers growing medicinal herbs. At Sacred Vibes, we continue to support our local farmers growing medicinal herbs by ordering for our apothecary when we can. In addition, we host a community herb CSA (community-supported agriculture) program where people can pick up shares every week to make medicine. I highly recommend this to those wanting a small number of seasonal plants to build their medicine-making skills.

Community gardens. Community gardens are the soul of each city. They hold medicine, the history, and the stories of the land. In just about every community garden, a medicine grower is a treasure trove of information. Spending time there gives us the opportunities to build knowledge of plants across cultures and for intergenerational connections. Arrange to work in the garden in exchange for some of the medicines we need. Ask for the weeds that some community gardens pull out because they are medicinal plants too.

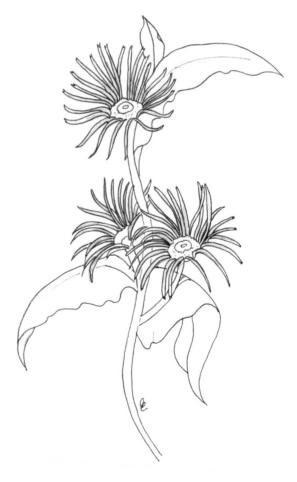

The Art & Practice of SPIRITUAL HERBALISM

ABOUT THE AUTHOR

Trained in Eastern and Western herbal medicine, Master Herbalist **Karen M. Rose** has dedicated her life's work to empowering individuals to reconnect to their own ancestral traditions. Over the past 20 years, she has created several outlets to offer her teachings and healing modalities to women, people of color, Black, and LGBTQX communities. The opening of the Brooklyn-based Sacred Vibes Apothecary, in 2009, was merely the beginning. Karen has now expanded her enterprise, opening Sacred Botanica and Sacred Spice, in 2020, two new locations in Brooklyn, to make healing more accessible to the greater community.

Karen's inspiration for this work began as a child in her native home of Guyana, where she was exposed to how African, Caribbean, and Latin American traditions profoundly influenced plant medicine and community healing. The legacy of these lands is the foundation of Karen's core values and spiritual practices.

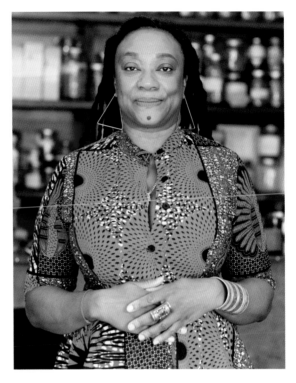

Regarded as a spiritual herbalist, Karen is revered for being the first to teach spiritual herbalism, plant medicine deeply rooted in ancestral healing and spiritual consciousness. Offering guidance to those on the path to finding the truth, she has trained over 400 herbalists through her Spiritual Herbalism Apprenticeship program as an act to reclaim their own health and offer healing to their own communities.

Karen's accomplishments include several in-house projects such as the Sacred Vibes' Annual NYC Spiritual Herbalism Conference, the 2019, 2020 Herbal Almanac, the Global Virtual Apprenticeship Program, the Spiritual Herbalism Apprenticeship Community, and the free Herbal Community Summer Workshops. Karen has been featured in the *New York Times*, *Los Angeles Times*, *Black Enterprise*, *Refinery29*, *Allure Magazine*, *Organic Life Magazine*, and Elle.com and has partnered with brands like BET and Squarespace. Karen currently resides in New York City with her three children, grandson, parents, and sisters. Her family is valued foremost, and all her work is supported by this firm foundation.

ACKNOWLEDGMENTS

Thank you to Spirit, my Ori, and my parents' Ori, under whose guidance I live, teach, practice, and heal.

To my grandmother, Eunice Bascom, thank you for being my first plant teacher. Thank you for your wisdom and the freedom to roam you gave me to learn from nature. Your lessons taught in proverbs light my way consistently. To my grandfather, Josuha Rose, thank you for being my guide in all the realms.

Thank you to my parents, Joan and Frederick Rose, for your love, support, and co-stewardship of my children that I may dedicate time to my community. To all my teachers, especially Kita Cantella, Tomas, Kalif, and Elder Malidoma, thank you for teaching me about what teaches you.

Endless thankyous to my children Lauren, Zion, and Shiloh, who share their mother with many. I love you.

My Sacred Vibes Spiritual Herbalism Community, a group of witches, brujas, and warriors, thank you for all your love, encouragement, support, and vigilance to our core values. You have taught me as much as I have taught you. Thank you for trusting me to heal with you. I appreciate you.

I invoke the blessings of the Essequibo Coast, where I was born and grew up. You have left an indelible mark on my soul. I am forever grateful for the life lessons that my homeland continues to teach me. And I am thankful for the city I have called home, Brooklyn, NY. You continue to demonstrate that herbalism can happen wherever you are.

INDEX

The Art & Practice of SPIRITUAL HERBALISM

sore throat
  echinacea, 184–185
  mullein, 38–39
  osha, 44
  peppermint, 62–63
  red raspberry, 106–107
  rose, 24
  thyme, 42–43
spasms
  chamomile, 160–161
  lavender, 134–135
  linden flowers, 25
spearmint: Sacred Womb Tea, 116
sperm motility: astragalus, 182–183
spilanthes, overview of, 188
splinters
  aloe, 139
  comfrey, 136–137
sprains: comfrey, 136–137
staph infection
  echinacea, 184–185
  garlic, 22–23
  lavender, 134–135
star anise: Immunity Chai Tea, 193
steroid use: astragalus, 182–183
strep infection
  echinacea, 184–185
  garlic, 22–23
  lavender, 134–135
stress. *See also* tension.
  chamomile, 160–161
  community and, 152
  echinacea, 184–185
  hawthorn, 18–19
  lavender, 134–135
  lemon balm, 158–159
  linden flowers, 25
  motherwort, 110–111
  nervous system and, 151
  peppermint, 62–63
  skullcap, 156–157
sunflower oil: 4th Chakra Heart
  Oil, 28

T

tension. *See also* stress.
  catnip, 163
  chamomile, 160–161
  lavender, 134–135
  lemon balm, 158–159
  linden flowers, 25
  passionflower, 163
  rosemary, 26
  skullcap, 156–157
thyme
  Breathe Easy Steam, 48

Clear Voice Smoke Blend, 46
  Garden Protection Bundle, 191
  Inspired-Sleep Dream Pillow, 166
  overview of, 42–43
  Thyme and Ginger Honey, 47
thyroid
  lemon balm, 158–159
  motherwort, 110–111
tinctures, preparation of, 190
tonsillitis: elecampane, 40–41
toothache
  echinacea, 184–185
  peppermint, 62–63
  spilanthes, 188
  thyme, 42–43
toxins. *See* detoxification.
trauma
  fo-ti root (he shou wu), 187
  motherwort and, 110–111
  oatstraw, 162
  nervous system and, 155
  sexual health and, 96–97
truthtelling, 76–78
tuberculosis
  elecampane, 40–41
  mullein, 38–39
tulsi, overview of, 162
tumor
  astragalus, 182–183
  echinacea, 184–185
  reishi, 180–181
typhoid: lavender, 134–135

U

ulcers
  aloe, 139
  calendula, 132–133
  chamomile, 160–161
  chickweed, 138
  comfrey, 136–137
  marshmallow, 66
urinary tract infections
  echinacea, 184–185
  mullein, 38–39
  plantain, 138
  violet, 139
urine, blood in: nettles, 25
uterine prolapse. *See* prolapse.

V

vaginal dryness: damiana, 112
vaginal steam
  Breathe Easy Steam, 48
  calendula, 132–133
  mugwort, 112

red raspberry, 106–107
  Sweeten Up Yoni Steam or
    Bath, 114
vaginitis: Plantain, 138
vaginosis
  garlic, 22–23
  lavender, 135
varicose veins
  cayenne, 20–21
  linden flowers, 25
  rosemary, 26
violet
  Face Steam, 140
  Five Flower Breast Balm, 117
  overview of, 139
vitex, overview of, 108–109
vodka: Protection Spray and Hand
  Sanitizer, 192
vomiting: red raspberry, 106–107

W

walking meditation, 30
warts
  calendula, 132–133
  dandelion, 84–85
water retention
  dandelion, 84–85
  hawthorn, 18–19
weight loss: fennel, 64–65
whooping cough: elecampane, 40–41
witch hazel: Rose Face Toner, 142
withdrawal from substances
  passionflower, 163
  skullcap, 156–157
wounds
  aloe, 139
  calendula, 132–133
  cayenne, 20–21
  comfrey, 136–137
  echinacea, 184–185
  lavender, 134–135
  muellin, 38–39
  plantain, 138
  red raspberry, 106–107
wrinkles
  aloe, 139
  comfrey, 136–137
  rosemary, 26
writing: meditative writing
  practice, 93

Y

yellow dock root
  Bitthas! Digestive Bitters, 68
  overview of, 88